GETTING
WELL
AGAIN,
NATURALLY

GETTING WELL AGAIN, NATURALLY

FROM THE SOIL TO THE STOMACH
by
Penny Kelly, N.D.

Originally published as *From The Soil to The Stomach* © 2001,
by iUniverse.com
Second edition *From The Soil to The Stomach* © 2005
ISBN 0-9632934-3-5 by Lily Hill Publishing

ISBN 0-9632934-6-X

Cover design by Penny Kelly

We are deeply grateful to the Weston A. Price Foundation for
permission to reprint the excerpt on hydrogenation from Sally
Fallon's book *Nourishing Tradition* on pp. 108-110.

The information, procedures, suggestions, and ideas contained in this book are not
meant to take the place of your physician. All use of this information is at your
own discretion. Neither the author nor the publisher will be held liable for any
injury, damage, or loss as a result of the information contained in this book. You
should consult with your physician before beginning any program of healing.

Nutrition/Health/Natural Healing/Holistic & Alternative Medicine/Organics

Dedication

This book is dedicated to my parents,

Hugh and Shirley Kelly,

who brought me up

with my hands, feet,

head, and eventually

my heart,

in the garden...

which led to a deep

and intimate connection

with Mother Earth.

Other Books by Penny Kelly:

The Evolving Human

The Elves of Lily Hill Farm

Robes: A Book of Coming Changes

Consciousness and Energy, Vol. 1

Table of Contents

Part 1
The Basics

1

Healing Is a Way of Life

THE BEGINNINGS were so subtle. First, there was a fatigue that rose early in the afternoons and would not go away. I was frequently aware that I was pushing myself to keep up with the people around me and with the daily schedule I had always maintained so easily. I stopped exercising because I was too tired to care about what it might be doing for me. The bathroom scales crept persistently upward, and I was 30 pounds heavier than I had been only ten years earlier. One day, in a fit of frustration, I went shopping and bought $800-worth of size 12 clothing because I was tired of not being able to reach, bend, or breathe in the shirts, jeans, and skirts that choked my freedom of movement.

My dark, curly hair, once a source of pride, was lifeless. I would look at it in the mirror and tell myself it was just my imagination that it was getting thin. I stopped plucking my eyebrows because they quit growing, and even my eyelashes were becoming sparse.

One spring day, my eyes burned and itched until I peeled the contact lenses off my dry eyeballs and put on the glasses I hated. The lenses were old, and soon it was obvious I needed an eye exam and an updated prescription. New glasses helped for a while, but over the next year my vision worsened slowly and steadily. I went back, got another exam and stronger glasses.

One day, while working in one of our small vineyards, I noticed that my ring finger hurt. Upon examination, I saw that it was bright red, rather swollen, and throbbed slowly unless I tried to bend it...then it protested with violent, excruciating pain. A few days later, I decided it must be a little arthritis, and when it went away on its own, I dismissed the whole experience...for a short time.

The following week the pain in my finger was replaced by an itch in the skin of my hands, wrists, and forearms. This was no ordinary itch. It was a deep, driving itch that caused me to scratch and dig at my skin even when I consciously tried not to. It would itch so badly that I would sometimes shake all over in an effort to discipline myself and resist scratching. Oddly, the places where the itching seemed worst showed no signs of rash or injury. I could not imagine why I had this maddening itch. When summer ended, so did the itch, and again I forgot about it. A year went by.

The next May, I went out to trim vines in the back vineyard. At the end of the first day, the elbow of my right arm was sore and painful. I tried to work the next day, but my arm hurt too much. I had overworked the muscles the first day and realized I needed to give them a couple of days to rest and heal.

A couple of days later, however, my arm was so sore I couldn't move it or my fingers. A month went by and now my right shoulder was as stiff and sore as my elbow and fingers. My back was also getting stiff to the point I could not bend or lean over at all.

I went to see my doctor who told me point blank, "You have rheumatoid arthritis and there is nothing we can do for it except make you comfortable." It sounded like a death sentence.

She gave me a prescription for naproxen, a painkiller also known as a non-steroidal anti-inflammatory drug, or "NSAID"[1] for short. I didn't start taking it immediately, but when the arthritis suddenly spread to my other elbow and shoulder, my knees, ankles, and the fingers of my left hand, I got the prescription filled and started taking it. Not until then did I understand the term "side effects."

---

[1] Pronounced *"EN-sed"*.

"Dry mouth" was listed as a minor side effect, and this was quite an understatement. Imagine trying to run across a freshly tarred parking lot wearing a pair of rubber boots in the hot sun. That image is similar to the effort needed just to speak while under the influence of an NSAID. Speech was not only slowed, it was often slightly slurred just from the necessity of having to take time to peel my tongue off the roof of my mouth or disengage the inside of my cheek from the teeth it was clinging to. Ditto for the eyelids, which required constant doses of my contact lens wetting solution just to allow the eyelid to slide over the eyeball while wearing my glasses, since contact lenses were now absolutely out of the question.

Before the arthritis, I did not like to bother with either cooking or eating, so meals were quick, often whatever I could find. Under the influence of the naproxen, I had no appetite at all. When I did eat, I felt slightly nauseous for a while. Pain played constantly in the background, fatigue was center stage, and I was now a non-performing act, too tired to do things as simple as walk across the room to get something I needed or wanted. I began to wait until someone came in the room and then ask them to please get whatever it was I needed, a trick of servitude I had always resented when others did it to me. If no one arrived to rescue me, I calculated long and hard about how much I really needed that item across the room. Often I was so drowsy that I simply sat, as if in a stupor. Other effects were heart palpitations when I did get up and move, constipation, a worsening of my eyesight, and sometimes even the feeling that it took great effort just to breathe.

In spite of the fatigue and drowsiness, at night I slept poorly. Every roll or shift of position triggered waves of pain that woke me up. In the morning, I would not feel rested, restored, or energized. Movement was slow and tentative; I needed help with everything, from carrying water to my chickens, to handling milk cartons, to opening the catsup bottle.

By midsummer, my right arm was in a sling, and I often used a walking stick to get around. The walking stick was a graceful thing with a bunch of grapes carved into the top, a gift from my uncle, meant to be decorative. Now it was an essential tool in any kind of movement.

At times, I caught a glimpse of myself in the mirror and was shocked at how old I looked. One day, while moving slowly back and forth in the garden, I noticed my bent shadow. That couldn't be me, could it? Other times I found myself in a moment of self-perception in which I seemed ancient and used up, withdrawn from the world and wishing it would go away. This was a drastic change from the way I usually saw myself, but I didn't – or couldn't – care. Pain was becoming the lens through which I kept seeing my life and myself within that life. Fatigue was undoing everything I had once been.

❖

One July evening after heat and humidity had steam-baked the family all day, my husband, Jim, asked if I wanted to go shopping with him in Kalamazoo. Although I seriously disliked any kind of shopping, the thought of being in an air-conditioned store changed my usual mind about such excursions.

In the store, I followed him about like a quiet puppy, content to be cool, saving my energy. He was looking at something near the book section, and I was leaning against the end of a display shelf when I noticed a thick book lying open almost in front of me. Casually scanning the page, my eyes fell on the words, "One side effect of aspirin and other NSAIDs that is often not mentioned is their inhibition of cartilage repair … and acceleration of cartilage destruction in experimental studies. Since osteoarthritis is caused by a degeneration of cartilage, it appears that, while NSAIDs are fairly effective in suppressing the symptoms, they possibly worsen the condition by inhibiting the cartilage formation and accelerating cartilage destruction." [2]

I was stunned. What was my doctor thinking in giving me something that would only make the whole arthritis problem worse? How stupid!

I bought the book, took it home, and read both chapters on arthritis. Then I got out the bottle of naproxen, opened it up, and dumped the medication into the toilet. "There! That's what I think of your medicine!" I said to the absent doctor as I flushed the pills away.

Over the next few days, I alternated between fury at our medical system and the pure entrapment I felt in having to rely on its methods of healing. These methods were not really designed to heal; they were designed to cover up the symptoms. As the doctor had said, they would make me comfortable – while I continued to degenerate.

---

[2] Michael Murray ND and Joseph Pizzorno ND, *Encyclopedia of Natural Medicine* (Rocklin, CA: Prima Publishing, 1991) p. 449.

Still, I was uncertain about what to do next. I had an aunt who had severe arthritis and was in a wheelchair. Her hands grew backwards along her forearms, a condition known as *ulnar drift*. She could not brush her hair or pick up a spoon. I loved her, but I didn't want to end up like her. She was in her late 70s and had seemed fine to me until just recently. Then, it seemed like her condition worsened dramatically and quickly. Thus, the first decision I made was simple…I was not going to end up like my aunt.

❖

That was the summer of 1994. At that point in my life, I had spent more than 15 years studying the mind, writing, exploring consciousness, experimenting with perception, teaching people to develop and use high levels of intuition, and working with researchers to understand subtle energies and the connections between science and the mind.

About ten years into this work I had become increasingly discouraged. Yes, I *was* able to teach people to awaken their intuition and to become extremely good with it. Often, they would astound me, as well as themselves, with what they could do after only a short period of learning and practice. But something always happened to get in the way of their continued development. They would *begin*, but they wouldn't *maintain* high levels of spiritual awareness and evolved practices. Since the expanded awareness and advanced practices were meant to improve everyday life, it seemed tragic that they couldn't implement what they knew.

"I'm wasting my time," I said to my husband one day. "They come out here, they awaken, and then they stumble…or forget…or get sick…or get caught up in some drama and fail to use what they have learned! At the critical moment, they stop believing in themselves. What's wrong? It's almost as if they don't have enough strength to maintain their own minds. If they can't maintain high levels of awareness and consciousness, how are they ever going to keep progressing? If they can't change their views of how and why things are happening, how can they ever *respond* differently to change their lives?"

For nearly five years, I had asked myself these same questions. But there were no answers, and I was coping with a growing sense of futility in my work. Maybe spiritual awakening, the development of intuitive abilities, a satisfying life of extraordinary creativity, and deep inner peace was not possible for the masses of humanity. I had just decided to do something else with my life, something that had more lasting effects, when arthritis appeared and took center stage.

One day, I was eating lunch alone at the kitchen table, staring blankly at the pile of mail I had intended to read while eating. Unexpectedly, the words on the top piece of mail stood out, "Nutrition as it is today does not supply the strength necessary for manifesting the spirit in physical life. A bridge can no longer be built from thinking to will and action. Food plants no longer contain the forces people need for this." [3]

My reaction was one of disbelief. "Nutrition?" I thought, "What does that have to do with anything?" The idea that nutrition could affect the mind or one's will power seemed absurd, yet I couldn't forget it.

Now, years later, in coming to understand the grip of rheumatoid arthritis and the dozens of other degenerative diseases plaguing us, I have come to realize *exactly* what nutrition has to do with things. After years of concentrating on the mind and consciousness, arthritis forced me to focus on the body and begin to understand it at a deeper level. In that understanding, I have been led once more to the fact that each of us truly is a body/mind system.

I have come to understand that people cannot maintain high levels of awareness or deep inner peace because they just don't have the energy to do so. They don't feel good. They aren't healthy. And very few realize that perception, emotion, attitude, and intuition are directly produced by biochemical conditions in the body.

My own illness thus served as a conduit that led me to re-discover what has always been true...that the mind can and does affect the body for good or ill, and in turn, the body affects the mind just as powerfully. They are equal partners in the body/mind energy system.

Since those days, I have made a commitment to learn what I really need to know to get well and stay well. This decision led me to discover much of what is presented in this book. As I have gone through this process of learning, nothing has surprised me as much as the fact that

---

[3] The words were on the back of a newsletter from the Josephine Porter Institute in Woolwine, VA. It was a quote from Rudolf Steiner's *Agriculture*, a series of lectures on farming.

so few of us know the information presented here when it is so vital, so basic, *and so interesting*. For me and my bones, for my husband and his lungs, and for others in our family with failing hearts, kidneys, or reproductive systems, this information has been the difference between healthy lives and lives spent coping with pain or disability.

Somewhere along the way, we realized that the commitment to good health might necessitate the willingness to change our way of life. Of course, it did become necessary, and the changes were much more extensive than we imagined. Therefore, I tell people right up front that a true commitment to health often requires that you let go of your ideas and beliefs about food and health. You must change the base of information you are operating from, and this ends up changing everything about your life. Almost without exception, you start by rearranging the daily routines that you engage in and end up changing what you eat, what you wear, the way your kitchen is arranged, your bathroom setup, your bedroom and sleep or rest routines, the work you are willing to do, your relationships, how you think and feel about money, your perception of real medicine, your yard, your neighborhood, and maybe more. In spite of the changes required, people get excited as they heal. They develop a new awareness of food and the other energies that we use to sustain us, and this can only be good for us and our planet.

For these reasons, I have attempted to present this information in such a way that you will come to understand the whole, integrated system – the body, the mind, your relationships with food, water, air, plants, animals, the Earth, and all of Nature. A little friend of mine often encourages me to "explore the nature of balance rather than attempt to restore the balance of Nature," and I will encourage you to do the same. This requires you to drop preconceived notions. Doing so often allows you to make the right decisions in the process of healing yourself. It is like the old saying about Caesar and God, but with a couple of modifications, "Give unto Bodies the things that are physical, and unto Minds the things of the spirit."

Although some people, especially New Age people, want to change the condition and health of their bodies using only their minds and attitudes, it seems quite obvious to me that most of us have not evolved far enough to simply "think our bodies well." And although it certainly helps to think like that, for too many people, no healing happens. We must take physical action, and that action must be appropriate. It has to be what the body *needs*. For if you are going to become well, you must learn to honor your body and its unique needs, not necessarily the way you were raised nor by following the latest food fad.

It is my hope that this book will help you understand why too many of us are getting sick, falling apart, dying early, or holding ourselves together with a regimen of drugs that leads to further dependence on heavier chemicals later on. Together, the illness and the chemicals we take for relief from symptoms produce fuzzy thinking and fatigue, both of which lead to an inability to see your whole situation clearly. This lack of clarity results in poor decision making around the subject of health and healing.

It has been the experience of everyone here at Lily Hill Farm that miracles do happen, sometimes even instantly, and it is my wish that, if you need one for your own health, you will come to understand how to make this miracle happen for you, whether it appears as a quick change or takes a few years to create. Remember, your body and mind must learn to work together, and once they do, you will discover you are the best doctor you will ever have! ❖

2
The Basics of Healing

IT HAS ALWAYS astounded me that we are not taught much about how to care for the physical body. Since each of us has one, this would seem to be quite an oversight, if not outright negligence. Most of the people I know have learned what they know about health care from television and magazine ads selling creams, potions, lotions, exercise programs, diet pills, cold and flu remedies, fast foods, and drugs. The message always implies, and sometimes states quite boldly, that the product being advertised will do something wonderful for a sense of health and well-being, a claim that is often pure marketing baloney.

Of course, these products would not be for sale if they did any immediate, overt damage, yet they have serious side effects that often create the need for additional prescriptions, and they distract us from what we really need to know and do to remain healthy. Thus, ongoing damage occurs while we neglect what our bodies require, and we continue thinking we are taking care of ourselves.

A great many healing techniques have been lost over the last 100 years, partly because so many of our old people have been cast into nursing homes along with their wisdom and knowledge, and partly because of our complete reliance on the medical profession and its emphasis on drugs and surgery. Drugs and surgery are so very important, but they should be the final step in the process of healing, after the natural – and much cheaper, more body-friendly – methods have been employed.

When drugs and surgery are the first or only choice, the result, for millions of people is a sense of helplessness when it comes to healing themselves. They can't afford the excessive fees that doctors and hospitals charge, and they have no idea of what to do to heal them-selves…I mean *really* heal, not just cover up symptoms. If you only want to cover up symptoms, that's all right, but the choice you are making will be expensive, the results will be limited and short-term, and you will find yourself enjoying life less and less. Eventually, you will be unable to participate at all.

When I was studying to become a naturopath, it was drilled into me again and again that, except for a dozen or so states in the U.S.,[4] naturopaths were not allowed to *diagnose, treat,* or *cure* people. We were not allowed to use the word *Doctor* or *Dr.* with our name, nor could we *examine, prescribe, administer, advise,* or *dispense* because these words have been copyrighted by the American Medical Association. For anyone other than a licensed medical doctor, these words were illegal to use in states that did not accept naturopathic medicine.

At first, this seemed to be a great disadvantage. How could we possibly work as healers if we couldn't diagnose and treat? However, as it turned out, there was no reason to know the technical name of every disease or every single, minute detail of the body's biochemical processes. Being able to give a technically impressive name to a disease does not mean you can heal it or make it go away. A precise biochemical diagnosis is only necessary if the intent is to prescribe a specific chemical that will suppress the exact symptoms and signals the body is displaying. Since we aren't dispensing drugs, it is unnecessary to pinpoint specific chemical sequences that characterize the processes of various organs.

Instead, naturopaths learn the basic systems of the body, how they cooperate and contribute to one another's functions, and what their basic distress signals are. We think in terms of the whole body/mind system and the lifestyle of the individual.

In states that refuse to recognize naturopathic medicine, those of us who have studied it are not allowed to "practice medicine," *but we can*

---

[4] States that recognize Naturopathic medicine are: Washington, Oregon, Ohio, Utah, Montana, Arizona, Alaska, Florida, Maine, New Hampshire, Vermont, Connecticut, Kansas, and the District of Columbia.

teach people how to go about healing themselves. Thus, I follow the ancient wisdom, "If you catch a fish for a man, you can help to feed him, but if you teach him how to fish, he can feed himself for the rest of his life." In other words, it is best to teach someone how to heal himself. Then he can do it over and over and even pass on the skills to those he cares about.

Except for accidents and unexpected infections, most illness and disease today is the result of a chosen lifestyle. Lifestyle includes – among other things – what you eat and how you prepare it; how much exercise you get; the way you handle your relationships with family and others; the amount of physical, mental, and emotional stress in your life; the kind of work you do for a living; how much sleep you get; whether or not you smoke, drink, or take drugs – both prescription and over-the-counter; your creative endeavors; your level of debt; your involvement in personal growth and spiritual awakening; where you live; the conditions in your local environment; and many other factors that make up your daily routines, along with the traditions of your culture.

As naturopaths, we are taught to think in terms of correcting the source of the problem, and we are shown again and again that the body will heal itself if we remove the irritating factors or supply the missing nutrients. The *body* is the great healer, not the naturopath or the allopath (*allopath* is the name for today's medical doctor).

If you go to see a naturopath, you will often be asked to sign a paper acknowledging that you – not the doctor – will remain fully responsible for your own healing processes. When you go to see an allopath, you are asked to sign papers giving the doctor full responsibility for your healing processes. This is not really fair to the medical doctor simply because he or she cannot force you to make the changes that will make you well again. If the entire burden of healing you is on the doctor, he or she is then open to being sued if the prescribed ideas and procedures do not work for you. It also means that you do not have to do anything different and that you're expecting drugs or surgery to remove the indications that you are living in a way that does not support and sustain life.

Although most people willingly sign over all responsibility for their healing to someone else, this non-participation adds to subtle levels of anxiety about whether or not the desired healing will take place. It is as if something deep inside of us knows that we need to change our lives if we want to heal. If the drugs and surgery don't do the whole job, and you were not allowed to be part and parcel of the decision-making process, the results are anger, accusations, and lawsuits, all fueled by the subtle anxieties that were generated by being left out in the first place.

Medical doctors are doing the best they can. Several of my close friends are MD's, and I have never met a medical doctor who is not acutely conscious of wanting to help others feel better and who isn't cautious in the attempt to avoid hurting or causing further damage. When something goes wrong, they agonize just like you or I would. Allopathic medicine is wonderful for a crisis, emergency, acute trauma, or other situation where "rescue medicine" can save your life long enough for the body's own healing mechanisms to take over. If it were not for the intervention of allopathic medicine, I would probably have only two children living instead of the four I gave birth to. One daughter would have been lost giving birth to my grandson. Another daughter would have been lost when infections got out of control. Thanks to the rescue medicine of allopathic doctors, I still have both of them.

Medical doctors seldom know much about nutrition, and yet a huge majority of the chronic illnesses and degenerative diseases they are struggling with are the direct results of poor and missing nutrition. To heal these, a different set of healing skills is necessary.

You can easily learn these skills. To do so, you must be fully involved with the healing process. To be fully involved means that you must be willing to do the work and to follow the techniques that support the body, not just take a quick pill and keep on running through life. You must also know that your medicine is sustainable. For your medicine to be sustainable, you must be confidant that what you do to heal yourself in one part of the body doesn't undo another part of the body.

When my doctor told me I had arthritis, she also announced that nothing could be done about it except to take painkillers. This is an example of very bad mental and emotional programming. It is also a perfect example of medicine that is not sustainable over the long haul because it does not address the source of the problem and bring true healing.

Although not everything that goes wrong in your body may be fixed to perfection, beware of accepting the idea that "nothing can be done about the problem" except to cover up the pain by altering your brain with chemicals so you can't feel the warning signs your body is giving you. The body sends these signals out for a reason! It's to notify you that you must do something different with your life if you wish to continue living. Covering up symptoms may make you feel better for a short time, but it is not true healing.

Understanding the connection between the soil and the stomach…learning a few detoxification techniques…coming to grips with the nutritional requirements of your body…filling in areas where your nutrition is lacking by using supplements…learning to trust the gentle, patient, healing ways of foods and herbs…doing a bit of exercise in order to increase the delivery of those nutrients to all areas of the body…practicing a peaceful mind…these lead to balance, healing, and the return of youthful energy and looks. *This* is true healing. As Dr. Richard Schulz often says, "There are no incurable diseases, there are only incurable people."

❖

To heal yourself completely you need to be able to create a complete and workable healing program for yourself. You have to know how, when, and why to incorporate the six basic aspects of a good healing program. These basic six are:

Food, Water & Air – organic, high-nutrition, whole foods consisting of meats, dairy, fruits, vegetables, and grains, as well as access to living water and fresh air

Supplements – Vitamins, minerals, enzymes, amino acids, glandulars, herbs, essential oils, flower essences

Detoxification – The Liver Flush, Colon Sweep, Purge, Castor Oil/Olive Oil Sweat Bath, fasting, castor oil pack, clay poultices, a variety of soaks and enemas

Exercise – Regular stretching, walking, yoga, and some physical labor or weight-lifting

Psychological/Spiritual Support – a person, family, group, or belief system that will encourage you to start healing and keep it up, even if things get worse before they get better

Home and Work – rearranging your life, your space, and your schedule to eliminate stress, carry out the various healing routines, and support good health.

A few comments I hear frequently from people who are desperately ill include: "Oh, I tried herbs already…" or "I take vitamins, and they really haven't done anything as far as I can tell..." or "I can't afford organic food..."

These comments usually come from people who try one thing for a few days or weeks, then jump to another thing for a few months, then skip to something else for a while, all the while hoping that they have found the magic bullet that destroys their problem. They want healing that will take little effort.

Let me say a few things right up front. First, if you have a catastrophic illness, taking a few commercial herbs is not likely to do anything by itself. It might help, but it's seldom enough. Ditto for the vitamins, especially since most people do not know how to take vitamins properly in the first place. A huge number of people do not realize how important high-quality nutrition is and so fail to make changes in their diet. Many people make an endless effort to avoid exercise of any kind, and they act like physical labor is beneath them. Lots of people feel helpless to do anything about their water supply, even though this is one of the easier problems to correct. Hardly anyone understands the devastating physiological effects of stress, and thus they tend to discount the necessity of eliminating stressors, especially if the stress involves a wife, a child, or a job. And almost everyone blanches when they hear the word "enema!"

If you have a catastrophic illness and you really want to heal, *you have to do everything at once.* You have to make the changes in your food and water, get the right assortment of supplements that will work synergistically, detoxify your body continuously, exercise lightly but regularly – not strenuously, just regularly – three or four times a week for at least 15 to 30 minutes, hold a picture in your mind of yourself in a beautifully healthy condition, believe in what you're doing as well as your body's innate healing abilities, and organize your home and work to support the food, water, detox, and exercise routines that will gradually become a way of life. ❖

3

An Early Pioneer

IN 1931, a small, energetic man with perceptive blue eyes was making preparations for a trip to Switzerland. Weston Price was a dentist in Cleveland, Ohio, and, over the previous decade, he had noticed a dramatic rise in tooth decay. Large numbers of people were suffering from cavities and many of them had lost 80% of their teeth by the time they were 20 years old. This was unprecedented! In the past, people had enjoyed excellent teeth that were perfectly formed and beautifully maintained with almost no cavities.

Like many health professionals of his day, Price was focused on trying to find the invading organism as suggested by Pasteur's discovery of bacteria. He was convinced that human teeth were under attack by some strange and, so far, unknown variety of bacteria.

Dentists were not the only ones dealing with an increase in health problems. Professionals from medical science, psychology, social science, anthropology, law, and other disciplines were noticing a steady increase in health abnormalities. Since 1907, heart disease had gone up 60%. Cancer had gone up 90% over the same time period, and the tuberculosis that terrified everyone was still spreading. People displayed an increasingly poor immune response, delinquency was rising, and there was a strange disappearance of creativity, motivation, and inventiveness in school-age children. Birth defects such as clubfoot, cleft palate, and mental retardation were up, as was infant mortality. Most disturbing were subtle personality changes and depressive character traits in people across the spectrum.

Working in his private clinic and research laboratory, Price, like his peers, methodically examined every possible theory and supposed cause of rotting teeth he could come up with. He searched diligently through his microscope for signs of unidentified and possibly injurious bacteria, but the result was the same every time – a dead end.

Meanwhile, at Harvard University, Earnest Hoonton had established the Institute of Clinical Anthropology in order to find out "what man is like biologically when he does not need a doctor, in order to ascertain what he should be like after the doctor has finished with him." [5] After thinking about this, it occurred to Price that maybe the problem was due to the *absence* of something rather than the *presence* of a mysterious pathogen. He began to suspect that the sudden, serious degeneration of modern people had something to do with what they were eating or perhaps not eating. Influenced by Hoonton's work, Price decided it might prove fruitful to examine the teeth of indigenous peoples who had not been introduced to the modern Western diet, which was based on white flour, white sugar, canned fruits and vegetables, jams and jellies, coffee, tea, and alcohol.

After writing to many major governments, asking if they knew of any groups of people within their territories who were still eating the traditional diets that had sustained them over thousands of years, he finally found one. The first such group was in the Loetschental (*let*-shen-tull) Valley of Switzerland. Once he found them, he and his wife, Monica Price, a registered nurse, along with a troupe of assistants, clerks, photographers, and other health workers, organized a trip to Switzerland to study them.

When they arrived in the valley, they found a group of about 2,000 Swiss men, women, and children who had been living self-sufficiently for over a dozen centuries and who exhibited some of the most extraordinary health in the world. The Swiss Guards of the Vatican, famed the world over for their amazing physiques and stamina, often came from Loetschental Valley or neighboring valleys with similar indigenous lifestyles.

The people were living in small villages at the bottom of the valley, with no cars, trucks, tractors, or even horse-and-wagon transport.

---

[5] Weston A. Price DDS, *Nutrition And Physical Degeneration* (New Canaan, CT: Keats Publishing, 1989) p. 17.

People walked everywhere they needed to go, carrying whatever needed transporting on their backs, and this contributed to both their excellent physiques as well as their strong hearts. Children spent six months of the year learning from books and the other six months helping with the tasks of daily life. Although tuberculosis was rampant all over the developed areas of Switzerland, there was not a single case of it in Loetschental.

In winter, these hardy Swiss stayed in the village tending their herds of cows, sheep, and goats. By early June, the animals began moving up the steep, mountainous hillsides, following the receding snowline in order to feast on the sumptuously green spring grasses that emerged from under the snow. Every June, the milk from these cows turned a rich, creamy yellow color, filled with vitamins, minerals, and butterfat. The villagers harvested this special June milk, making and storing large quantities of cheese and butter that was almost orange, so great was the amount of Vitamin A and beta carotene in it.

In the summer, they added a few greens and vegetables from small gardens to their basic fare, but on the whole, their daily diet consisted of thick slices of whole rye bread spread with butter, large slices of cheese that were as thick as the bread, fresh milk, and a bit of meat in stews or soups about once a week. Today we would consider such a diet a ticket to the cardiovascular unit of the hospital. Yet Price and his group found it was common for villagers in their 60s and 70s to be spry, willing, and able to carry heavy loads of grain or milk products up and down the hillsides without difficulty or fatigue.

The children of the valley played barefoot and without hats or coats in the cold air of early spring mornings or late fall evenings. They played in the cold water of mountain streams without discomfort and did not contract the colds and flu that were common for children who lived in America on modern foods. These Swiss children had almost no cavities, and Price found that only one out of three had any sign of ever having had a cavity at all.

Young people who had gone to live in nearby cities for a year or two around the age of 18 did show some signs of cavities, and a few had even lost a tooth or two, but as soon as they returned to the village and took up their former diet, the body created a hard, glassy, enamel-like coating over the cavity and the decay processes stopped completely!

Besides the strong hearts, excellent physiques, and absence of dental problems of almost every kind, there were other important differences between the villagers of Loetschental and those of people living in more modern settings.

The photographs taken by Price's research assistants showed that they had perfectly developed upper and lower dental arches. These dental arches offered plenty of room for all 32 teeth, which were always perfectly aligned. There was never an overbite in the two maxillary arches (the left and right maxillary bones hold the upper teeth and meet in the center, under the nose) or an underbite in the mandibular arch (the bone holding the lower teeth). The remaining bones of the face were beautifully developed with broad cheekbones, widely set eyes, and wide nasal passages allowing for easy, natural breathing with plenty of oxygen-carbon dioxide exchange.

Just as striking as the physical differences were the differences in emotional, mental, and spiritual character. These were a people who were peaceful; who had consciously decided that the development of individual character was more important than the development of material things. Children seldom cried or fought, they had high integrity, and their reserves of physical energy were astounding.

In sharp contrast to the people of Loetschental Valley were the people of St. Moritz. Oddly, in 1931 St. Moritz was already known as a health resort, and people from all over the world vacationed there year round, feasting on the most sophisticated and modern of foods. Price's shopping list of "modern foods" included anything made with white flour, sugar, jams, jellies, syrups, canned vegetables or fruits, and candy or confections of any sort, and to these the people of St. Moritz had plenty of access.

Traveling to St. Moritz in order to investigate the health and physical condition of its inhabitants and compare this to the residents of Loetschental, Dr. Price found that although it was a beautiful setting, every child in St. Moritz had tooth decay, with children under 15 having cavities in almost 30% of their teeth. In some children, an entire tooth had rotted away to the gum line. Others had abscesses in the jaw or evidence of scars from old abscesses that had eaten right through the cheek or the neck. Many were suffering from tuberculosis.

He was also deeply dismayed to find that the children of St. Moritz had narrowed jawbones and crooked teeth fighting for space. In many, the entire set of facial bones had shrunk, and their pinched nasal passages required them to breathe through the mouth in order to get enough oxygen. There were large numbers of goiters in the adult population, many forms of thyroid trouble, and a dramatic susceptibility to infections and diseases of all kinds at all ages.

After months of travel and study, Price returned to his clinic in Cleveland, armed with a huge amount of data in the form of photographs, measurements, dental records, information on personal diets and life-style, and food samples.

The following year, he, his wife, and the entire team returned to Loetschental for further study. This time, he began to suspect that the extraordinary good health of the villagers had something to do with the butter they produced from April through June, and when he left for the second time, he arranged to have samples of the butter produced in Loetschental Valley sent to him at regular, monthly intervals so he could analyze it carefully over the course of a year.

Although he was excited by his discoveries, Price began to worry that the superb physical, mental, emotional, and spiritual conditions exhibited by the Swiss in Loetschental Valley might be a fluke. He began looking for another group of people who had not been introduced to modern foods.

In 1933, he and his troupe of researchers traveled to the Isle of Lewis in the Outer Hebrides off the northwest coast of Scotland. In this barren land of gales and damp, they found a population of about 20,000 Gaelic people living on a basic diet of oatcakes and porridges, fish, lobster, crab, oysters, and clams.

Although the island was cold and covered with peat, residents managed to grow oats in the short growing season available to them. Peat was burned for fuel in homes that often had no chimneys. Instead, the smoke filtered up through a thatched roof, which was replaced every year, and the remains of the old thatch were carefully collected and used to fertilize the soil in their gardens. Houses were so smoky that it was common to see smoke coming out of doors and windows, yet this did not affect their lungs, eyes, or general health in a negative way, and there was *no* evidence of tuberculosis, heart disease, or cancer among them.

As with the Swiss people, they had almost no cavities. Their perfectly developed jawbones were filled with beautifully aligned teeth. They had extraordinary intelligence, along with peacefulness and a gentle, thoughtful character. They also had prodigious amounts of energy, which they used to work long hours, all the while enjoying the work itself.

As unbelievable as it may sound, nearly 5,000 sailors and fishermen would crowd into the port of Stornoway every Saturday night. There, they would sing, dance, and tell stories with never a fight or any kind of violence, and alcoholism did not exist.

I read Price's description of Saturday nights in the Port of Stornoway over and over. How was it possible that so many men could be happy and non-violent in that time and place, whereas we could not even put three sailors on shore leave without drunken excesses, fistfights, brawls, and competitive sexual aggression?

In tragic contrast to conditions on the Isle of Lewis, life on nearby Bardsey Island was much different. Modern processed foods had been introduced there, and people began abandoning their traditional foods and gardening practices. Bread made with white flour and smeared with jelly was common, as was canned fruit, candy, and alcohol. The result was the deterioration and swift death of almost everyone on the island. The cause of death was tuberculosis. When the government sent a second group of about four dozen new families, all young and healthy, to re-start the population on the island, they, too, quickly degenerated, all succumbing to TB.

Representatives from the health department went to the island to investigate, hoping to determine why the people should suddenly become susceptible to killer diseases. They decided that it must have been the smoky houses that were causing irritation of the lungs, which then turned into tuberculosis. In spite of the fact that the people on Bardsey Island had lived in smoky houses for centuries, health officials insisted that the people of the island stop their ancient, traditional practice of burning peat and allowing the smoke to filter up through their thatched roofs.

Those who followed the health department recommendations found that, without the smoked thatch from the previous year, their oat crop would not mature in the short, severe growing season that was typical on the island. Without a healthy, mature oat crop, their health soon faltered. A compromise was reached when the villagers finally agreed to move into new houses that the government had built for them, as long as they could continue to maintain the old houses with thatched roofs and burn peat in them all year, a solution that turned out to be both inconvenient and expensive. Yet, those who did so retained their health! And by analyzing the thatch, Price discovered it was loaded with nutrients and ash that gave a boost to the oat crop, bringing it to maturity quickly, a necessity in the short growing season.

With the visit to the Isle of Lewis, Price had found a second example of people following ancient, nourishing traditions and enjoying excellent health. Right next to them on Bardsey Island were the remains of those who had abandoned those traditions, only to suffer miserably and die early.

Each year for another 11 years, Weston Price and his group traveled to a different place in the world, bringing back evidence that everywhere the western European diet of white flour and refined sugar went, a sad trail of degeneration, disease, deformity, disability, and death followed.

Among the groups Price visited and lived with were the Eskimos and natives of Alaska. They lived mainly on salmon, fish eggs, caribou, groundnuts, kelp, a few cranberries, bits of sorrel grass, and seal oil.

He spent time among the Indians of Peru who fished along the Pacific coastline while growing corn, squash, beans, and other plants to combine with the seafood that was a mainstay of their diet. The Indians of the Amazon ate similarly except they also included birds, eggs, animals from the jungle, and yucca root, which is similar to potatoes.

The Melanesians, Micronesians, and New Zealand Maori lived on fish, crab, wild pig, fruits, and a few green plants. Polynesian diets were similar to this, except for a bit of taro root, which they made into poi. All of these groups had little or no tooth decay, extraordinary physiques, high levels of energy and stamina, and no degenerative diseases.

In sharp contrast to the seafood diets of Eskimos and those groups who lived in coastal areas, the tribes of East and Central Africa lived inland mainly on dairy products. Their diet included fresh milk products from cows and goats, some meat, varying amounts of vegetables, a few fruits and insects, and blood from their cows, something they considered to be of the highest value in maintaining good health.

During their trip through Africa, Price, his wife, and their research group had to be constantly on guard against dysentery, malaria, tick-borne fevers, lice, the tsetse fly and its dreaded sleeping sickness, as well as dangerous sunburns. Yet the African tribes who maintained their ancient diets were completely immune to such troubles. Neither were they familiar with arthritis, gallstones, ulcers, cancers, colds, bladder infections, appendicitis, infertility, abscesses, pyorrhea, or tooth decay. Only where the missionaries had succeeded in getting them to abandon their traditional foods had the African people succumbed to the difficulties in their environment or become subject to modern diseases.

After visiting over 30 African tribes on a 6,000-mile journey through their continent, Price wrote, "Their nutrition varied according to their location, but always provided an adequate quantity of body-building and repairing material, even though much effort was required to obtain some of the essential food factors. Many tribes practiced feeding girls special foods for an extended period before marriage (often for at least six months). Spacing of children was provided by a system of plural wives." [6]

Upon visiting the Australian Aborigines, Price felt they were among the most intelligent and skilled of all the groups he had visited. They exhibited the greatest endurance under extreme conditions and lived on fish, kangaroo, wallaby, waterfowl, birds, eggs, insects, and roots. Like the other groups Price had visited, they had minimal levels of tooth decay, no abscesses, no crowded, crooked teeth, and no degenerative diseases.

When he ran out of living people who were still maintaining traditional, pre-modern diets, Price studied the skulls and teeth of the plains Indians of North and South America. He also examined hundreds of ancient Peruvian skulls and skeletons, as well as other collections of bones and teeth wherever he could find them. None showed any evidence of tooth decay or what he referred to as "deformed dental arches" with crooked, crowded teeth.

In the end, the conclusions were unavoidable. Among the living groups he visited, wherever traditional foods had remained in place, people were healthy, happy, peaceful, and beautiful. He confirmed that before the advent of the modern Western diet, people were on intimate terms with food and knew specifically which parts of an animal or plant would provide the nutrients that prevented specific diseases. Again and again, he found that people went to great effort to assure that each generation was superbly nourished.

As for those who did not keep to the traditional foods, Price wrote, "In every instance where individuals...had adopted the foods and food habits of our modern civilization, there was loss of the high immunity (to many diseases)...It rapidly became apparent that a chain of disturbances developed in these people, starting immediately and rapidly

---

[6] Price, p. 138-139.

increasing in severity with expressions like the characteristic degenerative processes of our modern civilization of America and Europe." And the hundreds of photographs he brought back spoke volumes, certainly more than any words could ever say!

Everywhere he went, he gathered samples of traditional diets and compared their nutritional levels to modern foods. Each trip added to Weston Price's knowledge and understanding of what was happening to people and why degeneration was rampant.

At that time, it was already known that the human digestive system was able to extract and absorb less than one-half of the vitamins and minerals present in any given food. This meant foods had to contain at least twice the amount needed if humans were going to extract the minimums required for good health. When Price calculated the body's need for extra nutrition during periods of growth, pregnancy, lactation, stress, or sickness, he concluded that foods had to supply at least four times the minimum daily requirement in order to safely weather all periods of life without sickness taking over or degeneration setting in.

Price knew that a human being needed an absolute minimum of 680 mg of calcium every single day *just to stay alive*, and more to constantly repair and rebuild the body. He knew we needed 1320 mg of phosphorus, and at least 15 mg of iron. The minimums for magnesium, sodium, potassium, copper, iodine, and other minerals were also known or being studied. Thus, he had a useful yardstick for measuring the differences between traditional diets eaten by indigenous peoples and the modern diets eaten by the average American.

Analysis of foods in the average American diet showed them to be extremely low in vitamins and minerals regardless of where they were produced. People living on foods made from white flour simply could not eat enough to get the minimum amounts of nutrition even if they could afford to buy that much food. An entire day's worth of white-flour food contained barely 500 mg of calcium and sometimes only 300 mg. Phosphorus was present in amounts that reached 600 mg at best, and was often as low as 300 mg. These were far below the minimums needed for survival, and nowhere near the optimum amount needed for good health, high energy, and high levels of immunity to disease and degeneration. It was clear that modern foods were not supplying enough nutrients to build healthy bodies or repair them when they went down.

In sharp contrast to this, the average calcium in traditional indigenous diets was up to 7.5 times the minimum required. Phosphorus levels averaged 8.2 times the minimum daily requirement suggested by American nutritionists. Magnesium ranged up to 28.5 times the minimum. Iron was 58.2 times the basic need. Levels of iodine were 49 times the necessary requirement. The fat-soluble vitamins of D, E, A, and K were present in at least ten times the amounts found in the modern foods of the 1930's. And in every one of the traditional foods, there were significant increases – usually ten-fold and up – in the amount of water-soluble vitamins such as Vitamin C and B-Complex.

Because these high levels of available nutrition were missing in the modern American diet of processed food, the result, Price discovered, was an average increase in susceptibility to disease and disability of *thirty-five fold*!

Besides illness, cavities, and abscessed teeth, he documented case after case of physical deformity and immediate physical degeneration as soon as a family began eating modern foods. Mothers who changed from traditional diets to modern diets after having one or two children discovered enormous differences in those children born after the diet change. These later children were sickly, weak, and didn't look like the rest of the family. Many had club feet, poor eyesight, suffered from constant colds and flu, lacked strength, energy and motivation, and were relatively less social, seeming to feel and act like outsiders to the family.

The truth is, and always has been, that without enough high-quality nutrition, the body begins to skimp on basic structures. Jawbones shrink, become narrowed, and there is not enough room to accommodate all 32 teeth. The skull and cheekbones get smaller, and the face looks pinched. Often the middle third of the face looks "pushed in" and lacks natural beauty, or there is a jutting jaw with an underbite. Sometimes the lower third of the face is not developed, creating a receding chin and an overbite. Or the upper third of the skull doesn't develop, making the forehead recede, giving the face the overall shape of a ski slope.

In other forms of degeneration, the upper palate in the mouth takes on a high, narrow, tent-like shape, and when an infant sucks or a child chews and swallows, the push-pull stimulation of the tongue against the roof of the mouth does not happen because the tongue can't "reach the ceiling" of the mouth easily. This stimulation is critical for the development of the brain because the structures of the limbic brain, the pituitary, and the pineal gland are just on the other side of the upper palate and require the stimulation of sucking in order to develop fully.

In one amazing reclamation of human life and intelligence, Dr. Price worked with a Mongoloid teen of about 16 years old who was retarded, sexually undeveloped, and unable to function without constant supervision. Price operated on the boy's upper palate, cutting it apart and surgically spreading the two sides to create a wider, more natural shape. Within months there was startling growth. Regarding the young man, Price wrote:

> "With the movement of the maxillary bones laterally, as shown...there was a very great change in his physical development and mentality. He grew three inches in about four months. His moustache started to grow immediately; and in twelve weeks' time, the genitals developed from those of a child to those of a man, and with it, a sense of modesty. His mental change was even more marked. The space between the maxillary bones was widened about one-half inch in about 30 days...The outward movement of the maxillary bones (which form the roof of the mouth and the sides of the nose) by pressure on the temporal bones produced a tension downward on the floor of the anterior part of the brain, thus stimulating the pituitary gland in the base of the brain."[7]

This same young man's mental retardation dissolved to the point that he was able to learn to read children's books and newspapers. He then was able to get a job in another city, get himself back and forth to that job, and be a fairly self-sufficient human being in society.

Price also described and detailed other forms of subtle degeneration. A healthy chest and good lungs tend to be broad and shallow, thus breath moves into the bottom of the lungs quickly and is exhaled easily. A narrowing of the shoulders and lengthening of the chest leads to less-efficient breathing, analogous to trying to breathe through a straw. A deep, narrow chest leaves one susceptible to tuberculosis, asthma, and other pulmonary and breathing difficulties.

Similarly, narrowing of the bones in the pelvic cavity leads to great difficulty in giving birth, along with changes in reproductive organs that create numerous increases in miscarriage, stillbirths, premature births, and outright reproductive sterility. While on their trip, Price found

---

[7] Price, p. 368.

extremely healthy women on traditional foods who gave birth in bed in the middle of the night, right next to their husbands, without waking anyone! In contrast, women all over Europe and America were dying in childbirth due to complications of narrowed pelvic bones. When they succeeded in giving birth, their infants were weak and sickly.

Hand-in-hand with deep, narrow lungs, shrunken pelvic bones, and crowded teeth full of cavities went many cases of flat feet, clubbed feet, or instances where one leg was shorter than the other. Price found increasing deficiencies in hearing, huge numbers of children with poor eyesight, children with poor muscle coordination, sometimes cleft palate, or outright absence of the entire upper palate.

As disturbing as the physical deterioration was, the mental deterioration he observed all around him was even more upsetting. A number of his peers were dealing with burgeoning numbers of children exhibiting low intelligence, retardation, regular demonstration of un-social traits, an inability to learn in school, and a tendency toward delinquency, which often landed them in jail.

Price visited special education classes for slow learners, asylums and institutions for retarded and Mongoloid children, reform schools for the delinquent, and jails for those who had committed serious crimes. He noted that at least 98% of these children had the pinched, undeveloped facial bones and dental deformities that resulted from nutritional deficiency.

When he asked the director of the Ohio State Penitentiary if he had noticed anything special about the mouths of the inmates, the director's reply was that "there was a tendency for the tongue to be too large for the mouth".[8]

In a piece titled *Mental Deficiency*, A. F. Tredgold, as cited in Price's book, wrote:

> "The association of abnormalities of the palate with mental deficiency has long been recognized, and there is no doubt that it is one of the commonest malformations occurring in this condition. Many years ago, Langdon Down drew attention to the subject, and more recently Clouston has recorded a large number of observations which show conclusively that, although deformed palates occur in the normal, they are far and away more

---

[8] Price, p. 357.

frequent in neuropaths and the mentally defective. He states that deformed palates are present in 19 percent of the ordinary population, 33 percent of the insane, 55 percent of criminals, but in no less than 61 percent of idiots. Petersen, who has made a most exhaustive study of this question, has compiled an elaborate classification of the various anomalies found in palatal deformities present in no less than 82 percent of aments (mental defectives), in 76 percent of epileptics, and in 80 percent of the insane." [9]

In his travels around the world, Price had been struck by the health, peacefulness, intelligence, and sense of joyful self-responsibility that were so obvious in the groups of indigenous peoples he had visited. They did not have hospitals or jails. They had no need for such institutions and made sure that they continued to have no need for them.

Contrary to popular opinion, Price found that these indigenous people were quite aware of the rest of the world and of how that world lived. They were not naïve, ignorant primitives, wishing to be like us, going through their daily routines because they did not know better and had nothing else to do with their lives. They were wise and aware, and deliberately chose their foods and lifestyles because these ways created healthy, intelligent, peaceful people.

The women and men in native villages went to great lengths and considerable effort to obtain the high-quality foods they needed for themselves and especially for the young couples about to be married. Women went on special diets for a year before allowing themselves to become pregnant. While nursing their children, they continued this careful attention to nutrition. In many of the native groups, special care was taken to avoid another pregnancy until the mother had fully recovered from the previous birth, with a period of at least three years being considered as necessary for the recovery. No one wanted to give birth to a sick, troublesome child, a child who couldn't or wouldn't do his share of the work.

After years of studying and surveying people who enjoyed superior nutrition, comparing their mental and emotional conditions with those groups who clearly showed signs of nutritional deficiency, Price realized that personality, spirituality, and moral character were far more

---

[9] Price, p. 354.

dependent on the biological condition of human beings than had previously been recognized. He wrote:

> "Thinking is as biologic as is digestion, and brain embryonic defects are as biologic as are club feet. Since both are readily produced by lowered parental reproductive capacity, and since Nature in her large-scale human demonstration reveals that this is chiefly the result of inadequate nutrition of the parents and too frequent or too prolonged child bearing, the way back (to health) is indicated."[10]

Weston Price was aware of modern civilization's growing difficulty in getting good, healthy chicken, beef, pork, and lamb. He was always on the lookout for the possibility of providing high nutrition and maintaining superb health and immunity using vegetarian diets. In the same way that people were degenerating, so were plants and animals. Exhausted soil produced sickly plants with too few minerals in them. As a result, meat, eggs, milk, cheese, and other animal products not only contained fewer nutritional elements, the increasing number of deaths among farm animals due to proliferating diseases made these products harder to get and more expensive. The result was that many groups began experimenting with vegetarian diets. However, after years of research, Price wrote:

> "As yet, I have not found a single group (of people) building and maintaining excellent bodies by living entirely on plant foods...In every instance where the groups involved had been long under this teaching, I found evidence of degeneration in the form of dental caries, and in the new generations...abnormal dental arches to an extent very much higher than in the primitive groups who were not under this influence." [11]

In the end, Price reluctantly concluded that vegetarianism, as a way of life, was not sustainable because those who practiced this way of eating suffered from the same slow degeneration as those trying to subsist on the modern Western diet.

---

[10] Price, p. 7.
[11] Price, p. 279.

Recently, while attending a local conference on food, I was seated next to someone who was touting the benefits of vegetarianism as if anyone who ate meat was doing something dirty. I mentioned the work of Dr. Weston Price and the fact that he had traveled around the world for 14 years and not found a single group of indigenous people who thrived and maintained excellent health or lived to advanced ages on a vegetarian diet. I also commented that I had ended up with rheumatoid arthritis after ten years on a vegetarian diet.

The young man immediately protested my statements, insisting that the people of India had survived for years on vegetarian diets.

My response to him was, "Have you *seen* the people of India? They may be surviving, but just barely, and they certainly aren't thriving. The poverty and sickness there are devastating, and they don't produce the extraordinary bodies with the health and stamina that were once found among the Swiss people, the Eskimos, the South American Indians, or the Melanesians."

"But they are very spiritual," he argued, as if their vegetarianism was the source of their spirituality.

"Have you been there?" I asked him.

"No," he replied.

"Then what makes you think their poverty or poor health makes them spiritual?" I inquired.

He couldn't answer, and the conversation ended when someone gracefully changed the subject. However, it made me aware that a good many people lack the common sense to recognize groundless logic. India may be highly spiritual, but it is not because her people are hungry or have less food. It *may* be true that vegetarianism decreases aggression over the long haul because you have less energy to fight, but a decrease in aggression is not equivalent to an increase in spirituality. It *is not* true that eating meat increases aggression. The work of Price and others shows that it is *poor nutrition* that increases aggression while decreasing one's sense of social belonging, thus leading to the tendency for destructive behavior and relationships.

I recommend getting Price's book and reading it cover to cover. Even if you don't read it, just look at the photos. They tell a remarkable story all by themselves. What you will see in those photos is that here in America, the epitome of beauty – the tall, gaunt woman with a thin, aquiline nose, long narrow chest, narrow hips, slender face and features, complete with artificially straightened teeth – is actually an icon of physical degeneration. Many of our movie stars and models are a testament to the processes of degeneration and ill health in our country. The pictures in Price's book celebrate another kind of beauty that is just as pleasing to the eye, yet is based on superb health, something we have lost touch with in far too many ways.

Price's research in nutrition is monumental. Of that there is no doubt. For over 60 years it has stood like a beacon for those in the field of health, yet much of what he did has been overshadowed by "modern" science and advertisers who market foods to a public that pays little attention to nutrition. Perhaps Price's work came at a time when too few people were willing to look at the implications of what he presented. Perhaps what he was seeing and saying was too painful. Maybe it didn't seem real to those of his time, or there was nothing anyone could do about the way the world was going at that moment. Maybe they didn't have enough examples of poor nutrition to compare where they had been with where they were, but if we look back, a clear picture emerges of the forces and factors destroying our health today.

If you are looking for the way back to health, his work illuminates the path, and here at the farm we have discovered that there is no substitute for high-nutrition food. ❖

4
Poor Health Makes The (Business) World Go 'Round

CITIES HAVE COME and gone for thousands of years, and as the Industrial Revolution gained momentum, a slow stream of people began leaving farms for jobs in factories and life in cities. In America, the steady migration of people toward cities continued through the second half of the 19th century.

By the time the 20th century arrived, this slow migration became a flood. People began leaving farms by the thousands. They moved to the cities, took jobs in factories, bought food wherever they could get it, and adopted the white-flour/white-sugar diet because that was what was available.

Generation #1

Between 1900 and 1925, the first generation of Americans to be conceived by parents living mainly on a white-flour/white-sugar diet were being born in large numbers. We will call them Generation #1 because they were one generation away from the soil. As they grew, people like Weston Price and others working in the field of health began noticing problems that had not been prevalent prior to the turn of the century. Besides large numbers of rotting teeth, abscessed jaws, and narrow, degenerated bone structures, this generation was unable to resist even minor infections. Colds, flu, chickenpox, measles, and fevers were springing up everywhere. Although people often survived these milder physical diseases, they were increasingly vulnerable to the more serious diseases of tuberculosis, diphtheria, and pneumonia. Even when they managed to avoid the serious ailments, they were tired all the time and began losing interest in the active and self-sufficient ways of their ancestors. Worse, they began to suffer emotional and mental disturbances, and they could neither relax and sleep or rest easily and deeply.

As the health of Generation #1 went down, the number of businesses based on poor health went up. The rise of the dental profession accompanied the sudden rise in cavities. The profession of psychiatry made its first appearance, as did the need for mental institutions to accommodate the increasing number of people with emotional and mental disturbances. Orphanages were organized to take care of street children whose parents had succumbed early to the change in diet. Hospitals, doctors, and nurses began gathering influence and power. Chemists and scientists began to focus on substances that might improve health. And the sudden spread of infection, fatigue, malaise, and disease brought a wave of pills and potions, laying the foundations for the pharmaceutical industry to become the behemoth it is today.

Generation #2

Generation #2, born roughly between 1925 and 1950, was the second generation to be conceived and raised on modern foods. These children also suffered from cavities, loss of teeth, and abscessed jaws. In addition to crowded, crooked teeth that did not fit their mouths, these children suffered from constant colds, flu, ear-nose-and-throat infections, and some died from the childhood diseases that had once been considered only nuisance infections.

Over all, they were more susceptible to the diseases that plagued the previous generation, but deeper, more pernicious changes began to be evident. Serious birth defects appeared. Children were born blind, or deaf; they had misshapen legs and feet, and serious spinal deformities. Low levels of intelligence began showing up and retardation became more common.

As Generation #2 reached adulthood, they suffered from a vague depression, including levels of fatigue that left them capable of little more than finding a job and settling for a paycheck, rather than relying on their own skills, creativity, and ingenuity to maintain self-sufficient lives. Many who escaped being blind or deaf still found they needed glasses or hearing aids by the time they were in their 20s and 30s. They argued often, drank too much, and were willing to go to war. Once they passed 50 years of age, they ran into the long-term effects of the white-flour/white-sugar diet as serious heart disease, osteoporosis, arthritis, diabetes, tumors, and other difficulties continued to increase.

To accommodate this second generation of Americans raised on empty foods, there was an increase in the development of pharmaceutical companies, the appearance of the optometrist and the eyeglasses industry, the hearing specialist and the hearing aid, the podiatrist for foot problems, and surgeons who specialized in everything from removing tonsils and tumors, to replacing heart valves and hip joints. Associations were formed to help with blindness, alcoholism, or crippled limbs, while nursing homes began showing up here and there as the solution for dealing with the early wave of those who were falling apart and no longer able to contribute to society because of poor nutrition.

The easy availability of modern processed foods and imitation made new increases in population possible, and the dangers of this population explosion were ignored under the banner of economic growth for our nation. As the population grew, so did the cities.

As the cities grew, so did a variety of transportation, communication, and manufacturing businesses. As these businesses grew, still more people left the land to take jobs in these industries. With fewer and fewer people farming, it became harder for individual farmers to do the amount of work required to renew the soil. Crops began faltering and the result was the early appearance of the chemical companies producing NPK (nitrogen-phosphorus-potassium) fertilizers, herbicides, pesticides, and fungicides. Deliberately overlooking the fact that they were highly toxic, these chemical solutions were designed to push the soil to produce enough food for the burgeoning population.

Generation #3

Generation #3, the third generation of Americans to be conceived and birthed from parents living on foods without enough nutrition, was born between 1950 and 1975. All of the same difficulties that plagued Generations #1 and #2 also plagued this generation, plus a few new ones. Physical degeneration was now accelerating as the toxic chemicals introduced into agriculture began compounding the problems of poor nutrition. In addition to the cavities, loss of teeth, birth defects, poor bone structure, low immune response and its resulting string of infections, there now came a wave of allergies, asthmatics, and ADHD children. There were huge numbers of slow, remedial schoolchildren who had difficulty concentrating on anything. To make matters worse, eyesight problems made glasses necessary for thousands of 10- and 12-year-olds.

As the potent pesticides and plant sprays worked their way into the human metabolism, immune system function dropped to new lows and a subtle derangement of the glands that made up the endocrine system began to show up in people and animals. The endocrine system, responsible for producing the neurotransmitters, enzymes, and hormones that stabilize physical, mental, and emotional conditions within the body, began showing signs of serious disruption. Skin was suddenly full of pimples and blackheads. Thyroids became dysfunctional. Pituitary and pancreatic glands collapsed, adrenal glands exhausted themselves trying to cope with rising stress levels, digestion suffered, weight went up, and sexual and menstrual difficulties mushroomed.

Upon reaching adulthood, many found themselves unable to conceive or carry a child to term. When they did conceive, they needed Cesarean sections to deliver that child, and often the infants were small and sickly.

To cope with the problems and needs of Generation #3, we added a number of new businesses. The use of chemicals to fluoridate water was an attempt to prevent cavities, with no mention of its deleterious side effects on the brain. The toothpaste, toothbrush, mouthwash, and orthodontic industries became big business, as did the allergists.

The appearance of so many slow, retarded, and remedial children categorized as learning- or emotionally-disabled marked the beginning of the special education classroom, special drugs to "help" them, and specially trained teachers to manage them.

Whole hospitals sprang up just for children. Welfare offices proliferated to help those who didn't have the health, energy, or motivation to become part of the constantly changing economic landscape. Social services, juvenile detention centers, and jails began appearing in order to cope with the increasing number of youths who were poorly nourished, maladapted, and aggressive. Cancer research and treatment became big business. Cardiac specialists became kings. Psychotherapy was the rage for a time. We began playing with artificial insemination and test tube babies, cesarean delivery, and neo-natal specialists. And all the while, chemical companies and pharmaceuticals continued to grow.

By this time, Generation #2 was moving into middle age. Sadly, an epidemic of cancer, heart disease, diabetes, high blood pressure, kidney failure, stroke, serious depression, fatigue, and frustrating obesity marked this passage.

Meanwhile, the remaining survivors of Generation #1 found themselves unable to focus, think, or act sensibly in response to everyday reality. They were routinely shut out of the economic system and thus quickly lost any reason for living. When they became unable to walk, too weak to care for their homes, too fragile and confused to live alone or maintain their health, they were shipped off without even a second thought to the nursing homes that were now ubiquitous.

Generation #4

Today, we have a fourth generation of people raised on empty foods. Born between 1975 and 2000, Generation #4 suffers from all of the difficulties of Generations 1, 2, and 3. These earlier groups are today's parents and grandparents, and because the problem of poor nutrition has gone unrecognized, there is a dramatic worsening of conditions in all categories of disease and across all ages and social classes.

Infants are born prematurely, have dangerously low birth-weights, cannot breathe properly, or are born without an immune system at all. Two-year-olds have cancers, six-year-olds have arthritis, eight-year-olds have diabetes, and far too many ten-year-olds are bloated and seriously overweight. Children everywhere have killer allergies and asthmas. They suffer from digestive upsets and constant congestion of sinuses due to the body's ongoing efforts to dump waste matter from the system. There are continuous ear-nose-and-throat infections simply because the tubes that drain the ears have not developed fully. They are too short and at the wrong angle to allow drainage—all the result of eating food with no nutrition in it.

Learning disabilities are rampant making special education and tutoring not just a specialty niche but a major part of the education business. Whole schools have sprung up to cater to the learning disabled child. Other school systems count on "special needs" children for a major part of their budget money. Mainstream schools complain bitterly about the violence and social problems they deal with in their halls and classrooms while they continue to feed students the fast food lunches that are so devoid of nutrients.

Mental and emotional problems leave youth alienated, suicidal, or homicidal, simply because they are unable to bond. Jails are a huge segment of the low-wage economy in many states, and some jail populations are bigger than some towns and villages.

It used to be that by age 50, people were falling apart, but now those in their teens and 20s exhibit the same problems and a number are seriously dependent on drugs, prescription or otherwise, to help them maintain some semblance of everyday life. Young people of 14 years have heart attacks and die. Others can't sleep due to breathing difficulties. They fight irritable stomachs, irritable bowels, and irritable moods. Derangement of the endocrine system creates dysfunctional ovaries, prostates, adrenal, and thyroid glands. When the glands malfunction, we end up with all of the PMS problems, yeast troubles, urinary infections, weight gain, skin problems, hair loss, depression, and fatigue that signal the crash of the endocrine system.

We have support groups for everything from alcoholism, depression, and cancer to stroke, bulimia, and chronic fatigue. Whole industries have arisen to supply the sick and infirm with everything from special walkers and toilets to mechanical lifts that will lift them in and out of the bathtub or up and down the stairs.

The need for expensive braces and orthodontic bite correction is something every parent *expects* to pay for. Weight loss centers do a brisk business. And there is a proliferation of equipment – both small and large – that helps us manage and monitor everything from extra oxygen to blood sugar levels to fetal development.

Today, thousands of people in Generation #4 are sterile and unable to reproduce. Those who can't conceive pay enormous amounts for the chemicals and drugs that will force their bodies to produce eggs and sperm or hold onto a fetus.

As the number of sick has gone up, there has been a steady increase in the number of available doctors and nurses and plenty of financial opportunities for those in the medical field. The explosive rise of medical insurance and managed care industries, along with the now gigantic pharmaceutical companies has swept everyone into their pockets. The growth in supplements, herbs, and over-the-counter medicines has been nothing short of spectacular. And yet there are an number of people for whom the current medical system can do nothing, and that number is increasing.

The appearance of whole stores devoted to junk foods that are nothing but sugar and chemicals, all based on the demands of an ignorant, addicted society, have fueled the poor health phenomenon. And this year a sizable portion of our political energy was taken up with the issue of health insurance designed to deal with the problems created by poor food and its results – physical degeneration.

Generation #5

Today, those who can still reproduce are giving birth to Generation #5. These infants exhibit serious defects in their bone structure, organ structures, brain, and central nervous system. Of the last five infants that I know of born to friends, family, and acquaintances, not a single infant has been healthy and normal. All required extended hospital stays and continued, expensive interventions after being taken home.

When my second daughter was pregnant with her first child, she was several months along when she went to the hospital for an ultrasound. A month or two later she had another one. When she went back for a third one, I remarked that I thought it odd she should need another one. I had delivered four children without a single ultrasound.

To my surprise, she said she wasn't the only one getting ultrasounds; all her girlfriends who were pregnant had to have a series of them. I couldn't imagine why the doctors would need to peer inside for a look at the fetus again and again, and when I asked her why she needed so many, she didn't know, but promised to ask the doctor the next time she saw him.

His reply to her question was that ultrasounds were necessary these days because too many children were being born with oversized ventricles in the brain (a ventricle is a hollow area or cavity). The enlarged ventricles then filled with fluid, a condition commonly known as "water on the brain," which caused mental retardation and other developmental difficulties. The ultrasounds allowed the doctor to track the size of the ventricles, and if they reached a certain size limit, which was something like 10 mm, delivery was induced. When this happened, the obstetrician invited neonatal specialists to be present in the delivery room in case shunts were needed to relieve the pressure of the fluid in the infant brain, thus preventing serious damage.

I was stunned. The fact that today's infants do not have enough nutritional materials to build enough brain matter to fill the skull without leaving dangerously enlarged ventricles is further evidence of the degenerating condition of the human body.

As things turned out, my tiny grandson's brain ventricles did reach the limits set by today's doctors, and they did have to induce labor, complete with the neonatal specialists present. But he turned out to be okay, and there was no need for shunts or other intervention procedures.

❖

As I write these words, there are nearly seven billion people on the planet, and most of us are at least one or two generations away from any kind of involvement with the soil. We grew up running to the grocery store for food and believe that someone else will take responsibility for feeding us. We are so comfortable handing over this responsibility that it feels strange, unnatural, to even think about taking on this task for oneself.

Both media and government compound this sense of awkwardness around food, the soil, and Mother Nature by speaking of those who grow their own food as people who live at "subsistence level." They make it sound as if this is something pitiful and as if those who subsist on what they can "wrest" from the soil live miserably. The truth is that Mother Nature is extremely generous, and those who grow their own food enjoy a very full, healthy, and secure way of life. The biggest difference is that this way of life requires a different daily routine with different priorities; however, it returns a sense of capable self-sufficiency to the one who knows how to provide for himself.

A huge segment of our economy is based on ill health. Ask yourself, "Could the giant hospital complexes and their related medical businesses, the pharmaceutical industries, the jails, lawyers, and parts of the legal system, the social services industry, the nursing homes, and the biggest industry of all – the food processing industry – survive if we did not have a large population of sickly people to keep them in business?"

If you look around, you will see a painfully obvious truth: that our entire economic system is based heavily around the premise of sickly, weakened people who are too foggy to see what is happening to them. If we all took a sudden, serious interest in getting healthy, a lot of people would be out of work. This would include those who work in industries focused on food processing; the shipping of food; trucking; packaging; agriculture; over-the-counter drugs; prescription pharmaceuticals; the medical insurance industry; the medical equipment industry, including everything from x-ray machines to hospital gowns; medical personnel of every type including doctors such as heart surgeons, oncologists, orthopedic surgeons, pediatricians, and other specialists; nurses; dentists; orthodontists; lab technicians; optometrists; podiatrists; physical therapists; psychologists; psychiatrists; scientists who do medical research; workers who make prostheses and things like heart valves or other body parts; a good many social workers; a number of police and lawyers; many teachers and tutors; and the tens of thousands of clerical and accounting workers in all of the above offices or trade centers. We all talk about the rise of the service industry, and what we are really referring to is the fact that we all serve the gods of ill-health.

As a result of our disconnection from the soil, we have built ourselves an economy that is looking more and more like a house of cards. How can we possibly afford to get well if it puts half of us out of work? Yet how can we maintain ourselves as a peaceful, powerful people if we don't begin to get well and stay well? It is my belief that we can't even begin to approach the creative levels, the insights, and the stamina that will be needed to transition through this dilemma unless we do get well.

Because of our disconnection from the soil, we do not understand how critically important it is to maintain healthy *soil* in order to maintain healthy *people*. When I make this statement about healthy soil to groups of people, the response is almost always the same – blank looks and confusion. The masses of humanity no longer know or under-stand that we do not have access to food that will sustain human life.

Without a relationship to the soil and Mother Earth, it is easy to be ignorant of the fact that our soils are dead. It is easy to think that putting something in our stomachs is the same thing as nurturing and feeding our bodies. It is easy to believe that factory food is the same thing as real food. It is easy to excuse and overlook the fact that those who are raising our foods are spraying poisonous chemicals on them before they sell it to us.

So what, we think, if there's a little fungicide or a bit of pesticide in our fields and gardens... *so what* if there's no topsoil... *so what* if I eat the modern, white-flour-white-sugar-coffee-tea-and-alcohol diet? Everyone else is eating it. I have to make a living and don't have time to grow my own food. I don't even have time to cook any more. Food manufacturers can create something to eat as easily as the local farmer, and all I have to do is open the can or the bag to get a meal.

Unfortunately this is not true...and we do not know that we do not know. ❖

5
The Connection Between the Soil and the Stomach

MOST OF US think of the ground we walk around on as *dirt*, something unimportant, something to avoid walking through for fear of messing up our shoes or the rug. It's rare that people look at dirt and think of it as *soil*. It's rare that people think of dirt or soil at all. Since the majority of Americans are now several generations removed from any sort of relationship to the soil, news about soil is ignored as meaningless and irrelevant.

Those who have been in love with gardening for years often know "good dirt" from "bad dirt" just by look or feel. They are quite conscientious about adding old leaves and kitchen wastes to the garden plot in the off-season or through composting. Yet even among people who continue to garden, when it is finally time to gather those first peas or pluck that sweet, red tomato, any awareness of the soil and what it has contributed is eclipsed by the excitement of the ripening vegetables. Seldom do you find someone who eats a tomato and remarks on the quality of the soil it was grown in.

If something drastic happened to all the grocery stores tomorrow and we were all left on our own to feed ourselves, would you know how to get from the soil to the stomach and end up with something nutritious to eat? Knowing that food with all the required nutritional elements is the bottom line in staying healthy and alive, could you grow a balanced diet to get what you need? Could you do it year after year? If there was

41

trouble in the garden patch, would you panic and run for chemical fertilizers, weed killers, and insecticides? Or would you know enough to realize that sickly plants, invading insects, and weeds that outgrow your vegetables no matter what you do are the results of sick, faltering soil, and that chemicals only make things worse?

Few of us think of soil as being a living thing in its own right, but it is. We don't think of soil as something that needs to be healthy, and we don't worry much when it's sick, but we should. It's hard to find anyone who really knows much about the soil anymore, yet a major part of learning to heal yourself comes when you begin to understand the connection between the soil and the stomach. So let's take a short course on soil that will help you understand the most basic of truths: that healthy soil equals healthy plants, healthy plants equal healthy people, and it is your re-connection to the soil of the earth that will provide the foundation for your healing.

❖

Dead dirt is a combination of particles of sand, silt, clay, minerals, dusts, and miscellaneous forms of carbon-based material such as bits and pieces of leaves and twigs.

Living soil is a combination of all of the above *plus* the bodies of billions of living, highly active fungi, bacteria, and microorganisms with names like actinomycetes, streptococcus, staphylococcus, protozoa, nematodes, flatworms, earthworms, mites, beetles, snails, slugs, and centipedes. Together these elements constitute what is known as healthy, living soil.

Living soil has a structure to it – a crumb structure! This structure is made entirely possible by the presence of those billions of tiny living organisms, bugs, and insects. As these fungi, bacteria, bugs, snails, slugs, and other microorganisms go through the processes of everyday living, they excrete sticky substances as waste matter. They also die, then deteriorate into gooey globs. As we will see, all this sticky, gooey material is very important.

In the first stage of crumb development, the fungi living and growing in the soil put out fine, hair-like arms called *mycelia* that wrap themselves around an assortment of particles of clay, silt, sand, minerals, and decaying matter. This creates individually packaged "crumbs," each containing an assortment of nutritional goodies in them for plants. Once the basic crumb parts have been wrapped in the arms of the fungi, the sticky, gooey waste material from all of the insects and microorganisms acts like a glue that helps bind the crumb of soil together quite firmly. Once bound, the crumb will stay this way until it meets with the root hairs of a plant that then "unlock" its cache of goodies and feast on the minerals and other materials it contains.

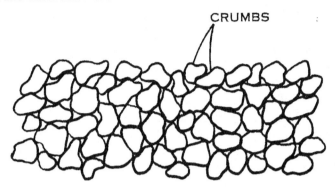

CRUMBS

SOIL WITH GOOD "CRUMB" STRUCTURE

These crumbs, together with the billions of microorganisms and other tiny critters, form what we call living topsoil. Topsoil should be at least five or six feet deep and have a complex honeycomb of air passages through which the roots of plants move easily in a constant search for nutrients, moisture, and minerals. [12]

A plant growing in good topsoil sends out main roots that descend into the soil at least three or four feet. Vegetables will reach down between three and ten feet, some herbs and weeds will work their way down 20 feet or more. Trees go even farther, as deep as 164 feet. [13]

From these main anchor roots, hundreds of very fine root hairs emerge, and it is the root hairs that do much of the work of feeding the plant. Each root hair extends itself outwardly, moving easily through the air passageways, searching the crumbs of soil for specific nutrients. When the root hair finds something of value in a crumb, it winds itself tightly around that crumb and emits a weak acid called *humic acid*. These plant-emitted acids react with the "glue" and other excretions of

---

[12] Deborah L. Martin and Grace Gershuny, Eds, *The Rodale Book of Composting* (Emmaus, PA: Rodale Press, 1992) p. 13-18.
[13] Bill Mollison, *Permaculture* (Tyalgum, NSW, Australia: Tagari Press, 1996) p. 223, 252 .

the microorganisms living in the soil, creating an additional assortment of mild acids. Some of these acids cause the crumb to break apart, exposing its valuable minerals and nutrients. Other acids then react with the exposed minerals, nutrients, and trace elements in the crumb, dissolving them into a solution that can be sucked up by the plant to feed itself and build the structures that will become the vegetable, grain, or fruit the plant was genetically destined to produce. [14]

When growers spray poisonous chemicals on their fields and gardens, *it is the microorganisms that are killed.* In spite of Mother Nature's extraordinary capacity to constantly restore herself, it takes only three years of chemical applications to completely destroy the life in a garden or field. Without the fungi and its mycelial arms, without bacteria, and tiny living organisms to excrete their sticky wastes, the crumbs of soil cannot form. The soil collapses into a compacted mass of packed particles. Without the crumbs, the numerous air passageways do not form, making it extremely difficult for roots to move through soil looking for nutrients. Plants must struggle mightily to work their way through this compacted mass. Their ability to find, dissolve, and uptake the nutrients needed to build themselves into good plant or fruit structures is greatly hampered, and thus, most of their time and energy goes into digging passageways through the soil instead of building healthy plants and an abundant harvest.

Plants raised in poor, dying, or dead soil are not healthy enough to withstand normal cold or heat, droughty periods, rainy periods, or the normal range of pests, fungi, and viruses that live in any healthy soil. These plants suffer from impaired function in themselves, their development is delayed, and the vegetables, fruits, and grains they produce are depleted or even empty of the minerals, carbohydrates, proteins, amino acids, and other nutrient factors that humans *must* have. The result is that *our* development is delayed and we become dysfunctional.

When the soil collapses, serious problems appear in other areas of life. Rainwater dropping onto healthy, living soil sinks in immediately and quietly. It does not splash all over the place nor does it create mud. Living soil with good structure does not stick to your shoes and boots. Instead, rain runs through the honeycomb of air passages and goes deeply into the soil. The deepest roots of plants get a drink, and the water not only dilutes the humic acids produced in the soil by roots, it also

---

[14] Martin and Gershuny, p. 16-23.

prevents a chemical burn that can be caused by nutrient or fertilizer overdose.

Healthy soil absorbs two to four times its weight in water before the saturation point is reached. [15] An acre of soil is roughly 208 feet by 208 feet, and the actual numbers multiply out to 43,560 square feet. Six inches of living topsoil on that acre will weigh about two million pounds and will hold up to 8 million pounds of water. Twelve inches of topsoil will hold twice that amount, nearly 16 million pounds of water. If the topsoil were five or six feet deep, which is what it should be in a viable soil system, it would hold up to 96 million pounds of water before it started to run off. Imagine, 96 million pounds of water in the space of about four city lots each 75' by 150'. That's 48,000 tons of water. Not only is this powerful protection against flooding, it is quite a reservoir of water.

This also shows why we are suffering from floods and mudslides in so many places, while at the same time running out of good, potable drinking water. We have destroyed our soil, and thus, much of our rainwater runs across the surface of the land and into streams and rivers, carrying precious topsoil with it. From there it goes to the sea where it turns to salt water.

Mother Nature has a water purifying system of her own, but rainwater has to sink deeply into the soil for the system to work. When the rainwater doesn't get down into the deep layers of soil, aquifers and springs dry up, and we lose clean, clear drinking water.

As of 2001, over 900 million tons of poisonous chemicals were being dumped onto topsoil each year. [16] These chemicals have added exponentially to the problem of collapsed soils around the world. Most fertilizers, pesticides, herbicides, and fungicides are so extremely volatile that heavy metal salts – arsenic, lead, cadmium, nickel, and others – are used to keep them chemically stable long enough to get them out of the bottle or box and onto fields and crops. We all know that poisonous chemicals are very bad for us, but the heavy metal salts are just as bad, if not worse. These metallic salts sink through the few inches of topsoil we have left and settle on top of the subsoil layer. Once there, the salts react with calcium carbonate in the subsoil in a slaking action that produces something very similar to cement.

---

[15] Dan Skow DVM and Charles Walters Jr, *Mainline Farming for Century 21* (Kansas City, MO: Acres USA Publishing, 1991) p. 35.
[16] *Acres USA* newspaper.

This cement is called *hardpan*. It forms a thick layer only eight or nine inches below the surface of the ground. This cement-like layer seals off the subsoil quite effectively and contributes to the water run-off mentioned above. Worse, roots cannot work their way past the hardpan into the subsoil, which often has at least some nutrients in it.

Roots end up confined to the top eight or nine inches of soil where they overheat on warm days. At 85° Fahrenheit, plants stop growing and begin to suffer from malaise or failure to thrive. Without plenty of water, things quickly become critical. In shallow soil, they soon use up all available nutrients and end up taking in large amounts of the heavy metals sitting on the subsoil as they try to work their way through it. The heavy metals are then incorporated into the structure of the plant itself as well as the fruit (farmers call everything *fruits*, whether it is a vegetable, grain, or an actual fruit). We eat the fruit and suffer thrice, once from the absence of nutrients, again by the presence of poisonous chemicals, and once more by taking in the heavy metals, something we will come back to in the chapter on chelation.

While this heavy, cement-like layer is forming a few inches under the topsoil, the exact opposite – a fine dust – is forming on the topmost layer of the soil. As bacteria and microorganisms die, the soil sitting on top of the land becomes a loose, lightweight layer of sand, dust, and silt. Without the sticky glue to create heavy crumbs, this fine, light top layer blows away in the wind, further reducing our ability to produce good food. When we dump toxic chemicals onto the soil, these toxins end up blowing away as well, polluting the air and eventually our lungs.

Over the past 100 years, our topsoil has washed or blown away to the point that its depth has been reduced to less than three inches. In some places there is only an inch left, while other places have none. A desert is essentially a place without topsoil, and this condition is spreading around the globe. Without living topsoil, plants struggle to push their roots through subsoil where they fail to thrive and soon die. Without a good layer of healthy, living topsoil, there will eventually be hunger and famine across the land.

When European settlers first arrived in America, they found virgin topsoil that was three, four, five, even six feet deep. Between 1800 and 1850, New York farmers regularly produced 150 bushels of corn per acre, and yields of 172 bushels per acre were not uncommon. Potato farmers were able to get 800 bushels of potatoes per acre, [17] all without NPK fertilizers, pesticides, fungicides, or herbicides. Today, we can get those yields only with heavy doses of expensive chemical fertilizers and lots of pesticides and fungicides to ward off bugs, molds, and mildews until harvest.

NPK fertilizers will make your plants look big, green, and healthy when they aren't; they're simply bloated and watery – thus tasteless! NPK fertilizers also produce a condition of overgrowth with too many leaves, stems, and shoots that the plant then has difficulty supporting, especially if the soil is dead or has started to collapse. By the time the plant tries to produce fruit, it is nutritionally bankrupt from supporting such a large plant and nothing goes into the fruit. The result is a crop that amounts to garbage, and that is where insects come in.

To understand the role that insects play in food production, it is necessary to revisit the periodic table we all studied in chemistry. Every element of the periodic table is surrounded by a vibrating field of electromagnetic energy. The pattern and color of this energy field is different for every kind of element, each as unique as a fingerprint. Using a device called a spectrometer, we can study this energy field imprint to determine if an element is present in a compound or a living system.

Every kind of matter, every molecule, every plant, animal, and human is also composed of and surrounded by a vibrating field of electromagnetic energy. When a plant has absorbed a particular mineral element, the frequency pattern of the mineral will affect the overall frequency pattern of the plant. The mineral thus becomes a contributor to the total pattern of the plant's electromagnetic field in the same way that a violinist or horn player contributes to the overall sound of a symphony. All of the frequencies of the various minerals and nutrients combine to help drive the plant's operation as a living system, and when complete, this vibrating energy pattern becomes a plant's electromagnetic signature.

Healthy plants that have access to all of the minerals and nutrients necessary to build well-functioning stems, leaves, flowers, and fruits radiate an energetic frequency that has a particular complex of electromagnetic (E-M) signals and tones. These mineral frequencies are the same frequencies that trigger certain genes into action or inaction, and it is critical that our foods be well-mineralized and nutrient-dense.

---

[17] Arden Anderson PhD, DO, *Science in Agriculture* (Kansas City, MO: Acres USA, 1992) p. xv.

Otherwise, we end up with genetically based diseases, and we spend millions of dollars trying to figure out how or why this gene turned on and that one turned off.

When soil collapses and the plant is unable to find the nutrients it needs to be healthy, it will be short on minerals and nutrients, which mean that certain contributions to the plant's electromagnetic signature will not be made. This causes the plant to radiate an off-color frequency and give off a different E-M signal and tone.

What you may not have known or realized is that the antennae on insects and bugs are exactly that – an antenna system for picking up electromagnetic wave signals. Not only do they work just like your TV antenna, they are built just like them as well.

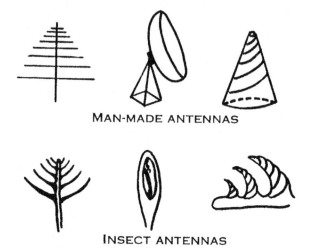

MAN-MADE ANTENNAS

INSECT ANTENNAS

(above drawing)[18]

Insects and pests use their antennae to pick up the altered electromagnetic signals coming from weak, diseased, or dysfunctional plants, then zero in on those plants to destroy them, simply because *that is the purpose of insects.* They are Mother Nature's garbage men, as well as her quality control team, disposing of inferior plants and plant or animal wastes in an efficient and timely way.

---

[18] This is not my drawing. I found it years ago in a book and never forgot the picture, but I don't know which book it was and couldn't find it after two days of looking. I felt it was too important to leave out, and I will be happy to give credit to the proper source if and when I find it.

Many people think that insects and pests will attack any plant and destroy it, but this is not true. When healthy and unhealthy plants in separate pots are placed right next to one another and their stems and leaves intertwined, the insects will ignore the leaves of the healthy plant and go after the leaves of the sickly one. They may take a few bites out of the healthy plant as a means of testing, but they won't destroy it. [19] Why not? Because healthy plants grown in good soil not only give off a different electromagnetic signal, they maintain a very high level of natural sugars in their leaves, stems, and fruit, and this is the magic key to pest control. For farmers and growers, this plant sugar is referred to as *brix*. You might think that insects and pests would be anxious to get to the plants with the highest sugar/brix, but this is not the case. Only humans are foolish enough to eat high amounts of sugar, another topic we will come to later.

Insects munching on plants with high levels of sugar quickly get a paralyzing stomachache and abandon the plant altogether. The high sugar combines with the bugs' internal chemistry to produce an alcohol in their digestive tract. This alcohol quite effectively knocks out the delicately balanced metabolism of insects and pests. Those insects that foolishly continue to eat leaves with high levels of sugar end up falling into the soil in a drunken stupor and become a tasty lunch for the microorganisms, bacteria, and other critters that live in the soil! [20]

In good soil that is fully alive and well-mineralized, a plant builds its structure and begins moving quickly to produce the high levels of sugar that will protect it from attack by insects. Brix can be measured with a pocket refractometer and may range from a low of zero to upwards of 25 to 30%. Once the brix in the leaves reaches about 14%, the plant will not be bothered by insects anymore nor will it succumb to mold, mildew, or rot. In a living soil with healthy plants, each kind of plant achieves this level of brix just about the time that the insects who favor that plant are reaching their maturity, displaying once more the marvels of timing and response we all have to one another in the web of life. Those plants that don't make enough brix by the time the first generation of insects reaches maturity will almost certainly feed those insects well enough to allow them to produce a second generation, and then the laggard plants will be completely overwhelmed.

❖

[19] Anderson, p. xi.
[20] Skow and Walters, p. 33.

Sometime around 1918, samples of soils from around the world were studied, and it was discovered that these soils were able to produce plants with viable protein levels of only 12%. The minimum level required for human and animal health is 25%. By the 1950s, soils in the United States were down to only 6% viable protein. By the 1970s, U.S. soils had sunk to somewhere between 1.5% and 3.0%. Today, they are certainly no better. [21]

William Albrecht, famed professor of soil science at the University of Missouri for many years, described a plant's struggle as one that strove to synthesize proteins and living tissue to support growth, provide self-protection, and reproduce. [22] The fruit is the plant's way of reproducing.

He pointed out that humans and all other warm-blooded bodies were also struggling to get enough proteins and that proteins were synthesized directly from basic elements *only by plants and microbes.* These plants and microbes then feed us. They also feed the animals that feed us.

"Protein contains nitrogen and nitrogen is essential to the construction of a new cell. A deficiency of protein, and thus of nitrogen, will short-circuit new cell construction and this signals the beginning of disease. In humans, this is called degenerative metabolic disease." [23]

The reality of this is now hitting home. There are only a few basic forms of illness. One form is infectious disease, another is degenerative disease, and the rest are accidents. Some have suggested that congenital birth defects are another form of illness, but it turns out that almost all birth defects are due to poor nutrition in the mother, and thus are a form of degenerative disease.

Degenerative disease is rampant in this country. Twelve-year-olds need hip and knee replacements, while thirty-year-olds need everything from heart transplants to lung and kidney transplants. Each generation is displaying degenerative symptoms at earlier and earlier ages. Almost every family I know has someone seriously sick, seriously overweight, or even terminal. Even those who are health-conscious get sick. Why? Because our soils are, for all practical purposes, dead, and even if we are eating fresh, whole foods that do not come out of boxes

---

[21] Anderson, p. xi.
[22] Skow and Walters, p. 169.
[23] Skow and Walters, p. 3.

and cans, those fresh, whole foods are seriously deficient in nutrition and, unless organic, also laced with heavy metals and poisons.

Over the thousands of years that people have been on Earth, whenever we have overworked our soil or neglected to renew it, famine followed. Dead soils and sickly plants invited attacks by hordes of locusts. When this occurred we simply picked up and moved to new lands. Droughts, or the failure of a group's staple crop such as potatoes or wheat, have been the driving factors in the continuous westward migration of human beings over the past several thousand years. Now we are at the end of the trail. We have migrated all the way around the globe, filling the planet almost beyond capacity with sick and degenerating people, dead soil, and polluted water. There is nowhere left to run, and the dreams of a Green Revolution promised by the chemical factories have proven to be more of a nightmare than a dream.

Fruits, vegetables, and grains that grow in dead soil are almost as dead as the soil they come from. Even when they look beautiful, they have minimal levels of protein, complex carbohydrates, and natural oils; they also lack minerals and vitamins. Worse, they contain chemical residues and other poisons.

We eat this stuff and wonder why we are sick or overweight. It's because the body puts out hunger signals when it is in need of materials for repair and rebuilding. Since cells are always dying and we use up many nutrients in the course of everyday living, the body is in need of a constant supply of top quality building materials – vitamins, minerals, enzymes, proteins, carbohydrates, fats and oils, and other nutrient factors. When you put food in your body, the body goes to work right away, breaking down what you have offered it to find the nutrients contained in the food. When it discovers there is nothing in the food, the body immediately calls for more food. This becomes a vicious circle because you have to eat much more than is healthy to get even a minimum amount of useable nutrition into the body. If you shortchange the body nutritionally for any length of time, you will find you are always hungry, always on edge, always unsatisfied, and driven to eat more. The result is stubborn and intractable weight gain.

People naturally try to figure out why their weight keeps going up. They blame the excess pounds on lack of self-discipline, not enough exercise, their metabolism, lack of time to eat right, laziness, or a bad thyroid. Often there are cries of despair that sound something like, "I've done everything I know to lose weight..." For most people, dieting becomes an endless circle of hunger, discomfort, denial of the body's call for nutrients, guilt when you can't resist that call, and shame over how you look (overweight) or how weak and undisciplined you are (low self-esteem).

Do not get caught in this circle. Constant dieting when you aren't getting enough nutrition in the first place results in low-level malnutrition, which leads to a lowered thyroid function. The doctor might test you for thyroid activity and tell you you're "low normal," but even a slightly lower thyroid function can result in low levels of the stomach acid that is required for good digestion and absorption of nutrients. Without a good supply of hydrochloric acid in your stomach, your digestive processes will suffer, and you will not be able to extract or absorb useful substances in your food. This leads to a critical shortage of nutrients that the body can use for repair and rebuilding. Because the body very carefully regulates what is in your blood, when the level of various minerals in the blood drops below a certain point, the body robs bones and tissues to get the needed supplies. Let this go on for any length of time and the result is osteoporosis and a host of other degenerative difficulties.

Constant hunger is the body's constant call for *building materials* that it can use to restore itself. When you eat, the body works for hours to extract nutrients, and when it turns out there is nothing useful in the food, your body has used up even more of its precious resources for little or nothing in return. It is like constantly mining for gold without ever hitting pay dirt. There are huge piles of useless waste material everywhere as evidence of how much work was done, but eventually the mining company goes bankrupt. The same thing happens to the body. It has chewed and dug its way through all kinds of food, waste piles up or accumulates in every cell and tissue, interfering with function, and efforts to continue rebuilding eventually go bankrupt because the body never hits the equivalent of pay dirt, which is the nutrition it really needs.

Picture a carpenter about to build a house. He has a life-or-death deadline to get the house built. He also has some of the supplies, but not enough. So he pours cement for the foundations but adds more water than he should to make the cement go farther. He has two-by-fours, but no insulation, a few windows but not enough. The doors that he ordered arrived in the wrong size but there is no time to return them and reorder. Installation of wiring is scant in a few rooms because he ran out of wire. Plumbing producers are on strike so he skimps on plumbing, and there was a shortage of ductwork for the furnace, so a few rooms have no heating or cooling. He does have enough roofing, siding, and paint, and so he proceeds to finish the house and make it look as good as he can.

The owner is pleased with the new house for a while but soon discovers that, although the house looks okay from the outside, it is uncomfortable to live in. Without insulation, he's too hot or too cold. Too few windows require more artificial lighting, but he's short on electricity because there isn't enough wiring. Poorly fitting doors allow drafts and bugs to get inside. The plumbing doesn't work right, some of the rooms cannot be used in certain seasons because they're too hot or too cold, and in a short time the foundation begins to crumble because of soft cement. Slowly the house falls apart.

This is what happens in too many bodies today. The "house" is crumbling. We are degenerating. To make matters worse, the body is not something you build once and then just live in. It has to be rebuilt every single day! When you don't have enough of the right materials to constantly rebuild, the result is a slow, downhill slide into degenerative disease and dysfunction.

When what you eat has been grown in dead, depleted soil, it will be dead, depleted food. Eating this kind of food leads to degeneration at all levels. Degeneration *is*...poor eyesight, loss of hearing, high blood pressure, obesity, heart problems, cancers, diabetes, thyroid problems, arthritis, asthma and breathing difficulties, allergies, eczema, cleft palate, bone deformities, club foot, kidney failure, the need for orthodontic braces, the need for cesarean sections in order to give birth, osteoporosis, aneurysms, dental cavities and orthodontic braces, high levels of cholesterol, psoriasis, and a host of other problems much too numerous to mention. When the soil collapses, we collapse.

It is time to recognize that dead soils produce seriously deficient foods, sometimes with as little as one-quarter to one-eighth the amount of nutrition as we used to grow when our great-grandparents were young. If we try to eat enough of this depleted food to get the minimum recommended requirements in terms of vitamins, minerals, aminos, and other nutrients, we have to eat huge quantities of food that leave us overweight and feeling sluggish, like the snake that swallows a pig. When these deficient foods are also laced with pesticides, herbicides, fungicides, and heavy metals, the degeneration process accelerates and becomes more vicious, more heartbreaking.

The time, money, and effort needed to restore our soils to good condition cannot be any more than the time, money, and effort demanded by the skyrocketing costs and burgeoning complexity of the hospital-medical industry. For those interested in a return to real health and high energy, top quality nutrition is a must. For a serious turnaround of the health problems in this country, we may all have to become gardeners for a while, or at least until those who produce our food understand that neither we nor they can survive on dead and deficient produce and meats laced with even the smallest amounts of poisonous chemicals.

Each time you go to the grocery store, buy at least one organic thing. If the store doesn't have organic food, ask the produce manager where it is, and this will let him know that organic food is important to you. If he says they don't have an organic section, just say thank you and go about your shopping. But keep asking! These requests will eventually filter through to those who make the decisions about what to buy and sell. It also is passed on to those who decide what to plant and how to grow it. If you can't grow your own food, you can at least have a voice in the food that is available to you.

As Weston Price once said, "Life in all its fullness is Mother Nature obeyed." [24] More than anything, before we can begin to heal, we need first to understand our connection to the soil and the food it produces. Once we understand this, we will be able to understand why we are in the condition we're in...and perhaps learn to honor the ancient, sacred path that takes us from the soil to the stomach. ❖

---

[24] Price, p. 419.

6
Trees, Earth, Water, & Air

I LIVE IN AN OLD HAYLOFT. A couple of giant linden trees, a silver maple, two red maples, a mulberry, and a Chinese elm extend their lacy boughs onto the third-floor deck that surrounds my loft. Just out of reach are a few river birch, spruce, cedars, pines, a magnolia, and a mountain ash. So close are these leafy neighbors that, at times, it seems I am living in the trees. Living up here has opened a small window into the tree community, introducing me to the domestic habits of birds, squirrels, butterflies, beetles, cicadas, moths, and several families of tiny organisms that create bumple-sized dwellings on the undersides of leaves.

Over the past ten years, I have become more and more interested in my tree neighbors and their daily lives. Trees are master alchemists who transform the gifts of sun, wind, and water into wood. Wood is a marvelous substance! We use it as fuel to keep us warm, for building boats, homes, garages, picnic tables, telephone poles, and everything else from rake handles to hairbrushes. Too often we think of trees as useful only after they have been cut down. But the gifts from living trees are far more important and useful than those from dead trees.

Viktor Schauberger, born in 1885, was a brilliant scientist who spent much of his life in the wilderness areas of Austria studying trees, water, air, their relationships, and the motion of the subtle living energies in them. He once calculated that by the time a tree is 100 years old…

...it has processed the carbon dioxide in 18 million cubic meters of air and fixed it as 2,500 kg of pure carbon in the form of wood

...it has *photochemically* converted 9,100 kg of carbon dioxide and 3,700 liters of water

...it has made 6,600 kg of molecular oxygen available for humans and animals

...working against the forces of gravity, it has drawn 2,500 tons of water in through its roots, up the trunk, and through the branches of the tree to its crown where it evaporates into the atmosphere for recycling and, therefore, purifying

... it has supplied one member of society with enough oxygen for 20 years. [25]

Trees are not just part-time producers of oxygen for us on this planet, they are major producers. The question that no one is asking yet is, "Who will dispose of our excess carbon dioxide and supply us with oxygen when all the trees are gone?" The ocean absorbs some carbon dioxide, but would it be enough?

Trees are a key player in the water cycle here on earth and another good question is, "Who will make sure we have enough drinking water when the trees are gone and the water table sinks?" Once again, the ocean is full of water, but it's not drinkable.

If we believe that the government will take care of these problems, or that we can turn our need for oxygen into a manufacturing business and let some commercial supplier sell it in return for money, our existence here will be considerably shorter and more miserable. It would be foolish to set ourselves up to buy and sell oxygen when Mother Nature makes it and gives it to us for free. We have already made the mistake of buying and selling mineral rights, water, and land when they could have been ours for free.

Oxygen is one of the most powerful antibiotics in the entire world, and already the amount of available oxygen in our world has gone down drastically. Ice cores extracted from glaciers at the poles were analyzed to see what the make-up of our atmosphere was in the past. To the surprise of the scientists, the amount of available oxygen in the atmosphere used to be almost 50% higher than it is today. [26] [27] Some

---

[25] Callum Coates, *Living Energies* (Bath, UK: Gateway Books, 1996) p. 216.
[26] Bio/Tech News, 1998.
[27] http://www.npl.washington.edu/av/altvw27.html

estimate that oxygen was as high as 38% of the atmosphere. Today, it is around 20%, even lower in some places on the globe, and those who have asthma or lung problems have a much more difficult time getting enough of this critically important element.

When I hear news programs talk about the destruction of the rain forests and its supposed effect on the ozone layer, I wonder why no one ever says anything about the drop in available oxygen and the increasing numbers of human beings who need that oxygen. The decline in oxygen, combined with the degenerative narrowing of noses and lungs, has led to a steep increase in breathing difficulties. Even more tragic is the increase of infections, cancers, and other problems, many of which heal when exposed to higher levels of oxygen.

As if building an environment that will support all plant and animal life, trees patiently create layer upon layer of topsoil, year after year. During the growing season, they send roots deep into the subsoil, and even into the deep rock layer. A good gauge of how deep the roots of a tree go is to look at how high the tree grows. Although some trees are shallower than others and prefer to spread their roots out laterally, there is often as much or more mass below ground as there is above ground.

Tree roots tunneling their way through subsoil and rock create a small mineral-mining operation. As with all plants, tree roots work their way deeply into the earth where they release mild acids from their root hairs. These acids dissolve tiny amounts of minerals from soil and rock and transport them up the tree where they are used to build the trunk, the branches, and thousands of thick, sturdy leaves. Each autumn these leaves fall to the ground, creating a fresh deposit of organically-mined minerals on the surface of the soil.

This layer of dead leaves offers fresh roofing material for an entire community of worms and six-legged "others" who make their homes under anything that provides a sense of shelter. Yet in a quirk of Nature, the worms and insects end up eating the house! Worms consider leaves to be an extraordinary delicacy and will make their way through a leaf pile with great relish, digesting the carbon-based green matter and leaving behind a trail of mineral-rich worm castings. Insects, micro-organisms, bacteria, fungi, and mycorrhiza breed and die among the fallen leaves, creating the dark, moist, living mass that builds slowly over time into a thick, luxurious, organic topsoil, known as humus. This mineral-rich humus becomes the perfect soil for plants, which then produce delicious, high nutrition food for us.[28]

This same layer of loosely stacked humus also works as a layer of insulation over the surface of the earth, keeping the roots of trees cool and moist, which promotes healthy trees and a good water supply. When the surface of the earth is kept cool and porous, rainwater will easily penetrate and begin to sink into the soil. This is the beginning of the atmosphere-to-earth-to-atmosphere cycle that produces living water.

❖

When I was a girl, I heard an ancient prediction. It went something like, "Long ago, God destroyed the world with water, but then made a pact with Noah not to do that again. The next time God destroys the world it will be with fire."

As we cut trees by the thousands, the soil heats up and dries out, the atmosphere becomes dry and dusty, the water table drops, and the timber turns to tinder. One stray match or lightning strike can turn whole regions into smoke and charcoal.

The world does not need to burn in one great conflagration for the old prediction to be true. All it takes is one drought after the next, followed by repeated fires in one region or another, until one day we look around and say, "Gee, I don't want to live there…it's too hot…not enough rain…nothing will grow there…too dry…there's too much danger of fire…their water is too expensive…they ran out of water…"

While listening to National Public Radio one day, I was astounded to hear a news report of a family in New Jersey preparing for a party, only to discover an hour beforehand that their well had run dry. They ran a hose from their neighbor's house to supply water during the party, but their shock at having to face this problem was obvious.

This may be just the tip of the water-shortage iceberg coming toward us. Even if we never have a full-blown water crisis, we certainly have a crisis of ignorance based on the fact that very few people truly understand water or that there is a big difference between mature, living water and dead, immature water.

Viktor Schauberger was the first to discover the difference between the two. He came to the conclusion that living water was born, developed to maturity, and sought to change itself into higher forms of

---

[28] Martin and Gershuny, p. 29-46.

energy. After watching the poor results from crops watered with what he called dead, "immature" or "juvenile" water, Schauberger spent years trying to teach people that water matures only when it is allowed to move through its full cycle, called the hydrological cycle.

This cycle begins when water evaporates into the atmosphere. Once aloft, it is carried by the wind until the temperature of the air cools enough to cause the condensation we call rain.

This rain then falls to earth among the trees, sinks through the topsoil, and moves down into the deeper layers of soil and rock. These deep layers of soil are kept cool because of the shade provided by the trees, and the cool temperatures help keep the soil porous. As the rain sinks down through the cool root zone of the trees, the water loses temperature rapidly at first. It continues its descent into the earth until it reaches a level where the pressure coming up from within the earth is equal to the weight of water pressure in the atmosphere. At this point, pressure and heat from deep in the earth begin to warm the water and some of it becomes steam.

The hot steam then binds with carbon in the soil and a chemical reaction takes place: carbon-plus-water changes to carbon dioxide-plus-hydrogen gas ($C + 2 H^2O \Rightarrow CO^2 + 2 H^2$).

Now the hot hydrogen gas begins to rise upwards again. As it pushes its way upward through the soil, it reacts with the minerals in stones, rocks, and other material in the soil, dissolving a variety of these minerals into itself and carrying these as mineral salts upward toward the surface. As the rising hydrogen gas reaches the cool zone maintained by deep tree roots, these cooler temperatures create an internal motion in the hydrogen molecules that is characterized by a left-hand spin. Known as *centripetal motion*, this motion is very magnetic. The result of this magnetism is that the hydrogen seeks out oxygen and bonds with it, creating water molecules that have an internal centripetal spin. Water with an internal spin moving in a left-hand direction is known as *mature, living water.*[29]

As this living water continues to move up through the root zone of the trees, some of the mineral salts precipitate out and are deposited in the root regions to become nutrients for the trees and other vegetation. In this way, trees and plants are fed via a slow-growth, mineral-rich system

---

[29] Olof Alexandersson, *Living Water* (Bath, UK; Gateway Books, 1996) p. 55-77.

that results in good health for the trees and superior quality wood for building projects.

Only when the water reaches the surface on its own and enters streams, rivers, artesian springs, or issues from other natural sources, is it considered ready to be used for drinking and irrigation. When kept cold and moving in rivers and streams, this potent and energetically beneficial water will remain alive and well. Those plants, animals, and people who drink it will maintain strong, stable, energetic, and healthy physical systems. The sick who drink it will be slowly returned to good health.

Schauberger deplored the pumping of "immature" water from deep in the earth to be held in pipes and tanks. He discovered that if water was pumped from the earth before it had risen to the surface on its own, it did not have the internal centripetal motion that was critical to life. Instead, its internal spin was *centrifugal* and was characterized by a right-hand spin, which he described as a "disintegrating, dissipating, destructive, or outwardly exploding force" used by Nature to speed the break-down and dissolution of systems to be recycled. This was just the opposite of the centripetal, magnetic motion used by Nature to attract and hold the particles necessary to build up life-forms and maintain their shape, strength, vitality, and function.[30]

In our present-day world, we do not allow water to come to the surface naturally. Instead, we dig deep wells and pump it forcefully to the surface. Once there, we hold it quietly in tanks and pipes where it is forced to stop moving and allowed to become warm. Warming has a very poor effect on water because it causes the water's internal motion to change from centripetal to centrifugal, thus going from magnetic (form-building) to explosive (form-destroying).

As water loses its natural magnetism and becomes dissipative, it begins to throw off its precious load of minerals and trace elements, which is why pipes and plumbing so often become clogged with mineral deposits.

When coupled with the other degenerative pressures of our time, water that is dead, immature, and dissipative contributes to our reduced life span of a mere 70 years. This is a shame when it is fairly well known that human life should be between 120 and 160 years. Scientists are now saying that the cells of the body have no known limits to their ability to continue living and reproducing.

---

[30] Alexandersson, p. 56 .

Living water turns out to be water that has matured until it acquires a left-hand spin with natural magnetism. This only happens when it is allowed to pass through the full atmosphere-to-earth-to-atmosphere cycle.

Once it has risen to Earth's surface, it must continue moving in the naturally spiraling ways that are characteristic of living water. Photographs of the inside of a drop of living water reveal extraordinary structure and order in what appear to be whole sets of currents, waterfalls, and oceans of motion inside the molecules, all of which the water uses to maintain itself while carrying the gift of nutrients to plants, animals, and people.

Immature water has not passed through the full atmosphere-to-earth-to-atmosphere cycle, and dead water is that which has been captured in tanks and pipelines where it warms and loses its subtle, life-building, centripetal motion. Like immature water, the inner motion of dead water is sluggish, centrifugal, explosive, and carries few nutrients to the living beings who drink it.

For many of us alive today, water is water. Our education has left us woefully unschooled in Nature's classroom. Said Schauberger, "Water in its natural state shows us how it wishes to flow, so we should follow its wishes." [31]

Those twisting, turning, snakelike bends that we see in every natural river course are the water's way of constructing its own path to maintain its high-energy spiral motion. When we straighten out a river, we ruin that motion. When we cut the trees along the banks and eliminate shade, water warms up and becomes lazy. Instead of spiraling along in a manner that literally and continuously excavates its own deep and narrow river courses with a range of temperatures to spur its motion, warm water stops spiraling, gets shallow and spreads out, slows down, gets muddy.

As pointed out earlier, when we cut too many trees from the land, surface soil heats up, microorganisms die, and the soil collapses. Falling rain cannot sink in deeply. Instead it runs across the surface, carrying topsoil with it. Most of that topsoil ends up in the river, choking the waterways and filling in the channel the river is constantly trying to dig out for itself.

The bottom line is that when water does not sink deeply into the earth, we end up with water that has not passed through the entire water

---

[31] Alexandersson, p. 34.

cycle. The water table slowly drops, and there is less fresh water to drink. We end up drinking dead water with centrifugal energies that explode our good health. We water the plants in our garden with dead water and wonder why we're fighting fungus and mildew all season long. The missing minerals and energies that should have been in the water contribute to plants that are structurally weak. In the same way that we use calcium, magnesium, iron, and other minerals to build good, strong bones, plants use the same minerals to build strong, healthy leaves and stems. Without these minerals, they are highly susceptible to the same decays, molds, mildews, and rots that we are.

In the same way that we have been ignorant of the fact that the soil is alive, most of us don't know that water is alive. We didn't know that when we captured water out of the rivers and underground reservoirs, forcing it into pipes, tanks, and drainage ditches, that we were interfering with the internal energies it used to sustain itself and us. We didn't know about water's maturity and powerful abilities to build living forms.

Schauberger predicted the day when a barrel of water would sell for more than a barrel of oil, and he was right. These days a 55-gallon barrel of oil runs between $65 and $100. We pay between $1.50 and $4.00 for a quart of good mineral water. That puts the cost of the water somewhere between $330.00 and $880.00 per barrel!

Schauberger's favorite saying points the path for all of us: "Study Nature and then copy Her." [32]

❖

When my husband and I were first married, we had a beautiful chalet in the forests of northern Michigan. When the wind blew with quite a bit of force, you could hear it, and you could see the tops of the tallest trees moving, but on the ground the air was quiet and still.

When it rained, it had to rain long enough and hard enough for water to get to the "through-fall" stage where it actually reached the ground because so much was collected by the trees first. Mud puddles were rare because the soil was so absorbent, and I thought it was my imagination that things rarely got dusty. Later, when I began to study trees, I discovered that 3,000 feet inside the edge of a forest, the trees will have cleaned, sifted, and filtered the air to a sparkling, dust-free

---

[32] Alexandersson, p. 34.

state. This, combined with the cool, moist, oxygenated air, made it easier to breathe. My husband's asthma eased greatly, fatigue disappeared, and we were left feeling energized.

When we bought our farm in 1987, there were woefully few trees on the property, which had been farmed for years and sprayed half to death. Each year, we plant at least a dozen more trees in an attempt to restore our little corner of the earth. Each year since 1988, it has gotten a little hotter and drier. Thus, we celebrate each tree that survives, encouraging it to keep growing with doses of living water.

A full-size tree has been estimated to have as many as 100,000 growing tips on it, and research now suggests that each tip is a unique genetic individual. Cutting a branch off a *deciduous* tree in order to graft it or re-root it elsewhere has occasionally resulted in the growth of an *evergreen* tree. When a mammal produces seed, all the seeds come from within that one body. But when a tree produces seed, each seed comes from a different flower – which may have picked up genes from something in the air, the rain, something carried on a visiting insect, or perhaps it was responding to a unique set of microclimate conditions on one side of a tree. It is possible that a tree is a collection of compatible genetic individuals, each with a set of persistent characteristics differing from place to place on the tree and responding to changing energies and other stimuli. Cutting down trees in wholesale fashion destroys 100,000 possibilities for genetic adaptation with every tree that loses to the saw. [33]

If you look back in time just a bit, you will see that for thousands of years, our leafy allies stood quietly on mountainsides, holding on to the soil, keeping it from sliding away and piling itself onto villages below. Trees that didn't mind wet feet stood at the edges of the sea to catch waves that came with great storms. Those trees kept the land from being washed away. Great swamps formed at land's end and whole trees went down in them, becoming huge masses of absorbent carbon to hold water. This created unique neighborhoods for a whole new assortment of flying, crawling, swimming creatures, and an even more varied collection of water-loving plants, flowers, vines, and bushes.

Today, mudslides and floods are a year-round problem. We build dams and dikes for billions of dollars and tell ourselves we have "created jobs," when a more accurate perception is that we have only ruined Mother Nature and made more work for ourselves. When it comes right down to it, we could not find enough men and money to do the work that

---

[33] Mollison, p. 139.

trees do, and if we could, the quality of their work would not even come close to the expertise and quality of the work done by trees.

When I drive along certain streets just outside our community, there are huge residential lots with big, expensive houses on them. They have $10,000 worth of landscaping around the foundation and deck of these houses, with a few young trees planted in the yard, some deciduous and some evergreen.

The evergreen trees, which collect and then radiate heat, are often clustered around the air conditioning unit because the wide branches at the base of the tree hide the ugly unit from the street or the neighbors. It would make more sense to shade the compressor unit with a tree that offers shade, rather than one that radiates the heat right back at the compressor, but too often we do things only for looks.

On any hot, summer day the sprinkler system in these yards will be on, watering trees, flowers, and bushes, and it is clear we no longer know or care what young trees need. Trees are extremely sensitive to light and heat. In the forest, young trees grow to maturity under the shady protection of the mother trees. They are healthiest, strongest, straightest, and produce the best wood when grown slowly in cool, diffuse light. Their annual tree rings will be small and close together, which helps the wood maintain its shape when turned into lumber. Their trunks are wide at the bottom and taper nicely to the top, a shape that is essential for the tree's good health. Those with smooth bark prefer dim light and will often be found in the center of the forest. Those with rough or shaggy bark will be okay in the sun at the edge of the tree line.

When shade-loving trees are grown in full sun, their temperature rises, and this is equivalent to being in a "fevered" state. Their internal metabolism is disrupted, and they may be unable to fight invasion by parasites, fungi, or bacteria.

When trees sitting in full sun are watered with dead or immature water, they grow too quickly and their annual rings become widely spaced and corky instead of tight and compact. This results in a weak tree that is not only susceptible to disease, it may suffer violent damage, the loss of limbs, or even uprooting during periods of high wind or ice storms.

When grown in the sun, trunks tend to be straight, round, and cylindrical all the way to the top rather than tapering. Yet this tapering shape is the key form by which a tree maintains the high-energy metabolism it needs to continue developing, to transport minerals and nutrients all the way up, and to stay healthy throughout its life.

Industry prefers the quick-growing, cylindrical trunks of modern tree farms, but much of the wood is weak, twists out of shape when dried in the kiln, and rots too quickly at the lumberyard. It is ironic that a tree that has stood outside through winter snows, summer rains, spring winds, and numerous temperature changes must now be sheltered from all these once it gets to the lumberyard lest it rot before it is incorporated into a house and sheltered by aluminum or vinyl siding.

My mother worked in a lumberyard when I was a girl, and I remember running and climbing among huge piles of pine and oak that sat outside all year. Nowadays, if you leave piles of wood outside for any length of time, they curl up enough to be suitable only for the bottoms of rocking chairs.

Besides its preference for light and shade, each tree has a personality expressed in its patterns of shape, color, the texture of its bark, and personal rhythms for leafing out, flowering, or closing down as winter approaches. Each has its own sound, expressed by the movement of wind through branches that are plentiful, sparse, tightly compacted, or widely spread.

The trees outside my loft also have a language of sounds by which they send messages to those who are listening. There is the soft hissing sound that is heard at the start of a light summer shower when you can't yet see or feel the first drops of rain. There is the soft soughing sound that pines make when the winds of spring arrive and there will be no more severe winter storms. Once in a while, they have great roaring conversations with a gale wind who comes by to prune dead or weakened limbs. I also overhear shimmery, rustling conversations among them, sometimes strain to hear their whispers, and at times, am in awe of their towering silence. How can anything be so huge and so quiet, like a patient giant standing outside my door?

Once I had a conversation with a tree. I asked if it had anything to add to what I was writing about it.

"Yes," it replied, "the very page from which your words rise is a transformed tree, sacrificed to make paper. Why don't you people learn to communicate and leave us alone?"

Needless to say, my shock was complete. Suddenly, I was aware that every piece of paper, every book, card, or letter expressed the silent voice of the tree from which it had been made. The tree's thoughts, hopes, and presence were woven among the words we placed upon that paper. How many trees had given their lives that we might send letters, invoices, greeting cards, newspapers, and advertisements back and forth and then into the wastebasket?

When I go into the city, I am appalled at the thin, sickly-looking trees cemented in place along the edges of sidewalks or marooned in an ocean of asphalt laid down to make a parking lot.

"Look at those poor trees," I once said to a friend. "Why did they even bother to plant them in this kind of environment?"

"People like trees," she said, "they like a little greenery."

"But what about the trees?" I asked.

"What about them?" she replied with a small shrug. It was an eloquent testament to the divorce that took place between humans and Nature generations ago, and it also points in the direction we must begin to move. As Schauberger once believed, and I now agree, we will only be able to achieve stability in the world if we immediately return to honoring our soil, water, and forests.

Sometimes, I look out across the field and see the ghosts of lost trees, thousands of them. The place I live in – an old barn – was built with a framework of tall, strong tree trunks. The bark is still on some of them. I wonder if the family who built this barn gave any thought to replacing the sixteen trees they cut from the woods and planted in cement to stand for at least a hundred years holding up the small forest of rafters, roof boards, and siding that makes this a barn.

Whether they did or not, it is time for us to begin thinking about such things. Umbrellas in a light rain...specialists in chemical manufacture...modifiers of the wind...endposts on a hammock... monkeybars to a five-year-old...landlord to 10,000 "others"...the tree is a world in itself, a living being that literally makes it possible for us to live, breathe, and share this time and place with it and each other. ❖

Part 2

Real Food

7

Food for the Masses

FOOD, THE MOST BASIC of necessities, seems to be everywhere in America. Everywhere you go you see it, or at least the suggestion that you can get it quickly and easily, with little work or distraction. This illusion of plenty is exactly that, an illusion, existing mostly in First World countries. In the entire history of humans upon the earth, no other single factor has commanded such continual reckoning with as the issue of food.

For thousands of years, we were pulled to the soil, anchored by it, yoked to it. Favorite plots of ground were chosen along big rivers that flooded every spring, depositing an annual dose of natural fertilizers in the form of silts that left the soil rich and fertile. If the river changed course or the land became exhausted, we moved on to a fresh place, leaving the old location fallow and allowing it to renew itself.

Back then, we did not have complex scientific descriptions of what went on in the soil, but even in our less scientific stages we knew the soil was alive. We sang to it, danced over it, sweet-talking, coaxing it to produce, and it did because it was alive and healthy!

Early men and women learned quickly that healthy, nourishing food brimming with nutrition was the key to survival and their ability to reproduce without problems. Food wasn't just something to put in the stomach or titillate the tongue. Those without superior nutrition did not survive. Without high levels of nutrition, babies were born weak or deformed, young people became irritable and unwilling or unable to participate in the work that was necessary to keep the group alive. Adults succumbed too soon to difficult conditions, illness, or infections. Whole settlements arose then disappeared when high quality nutrition was unavailable.

Those who survived followed daily routines designed to assure themselves of the best nature had to offer in terms of nutrients. The goal was to maintain radiant health. No tribe could be hampered by a child that needed constant doctoring. Nomadic families could not afford to haul around members who couldn't keep pace with them, and no group could afford to constantly support members who did not contribute to the group itself. More importantly, no one wanted to *be* the sick one, the cripple, or the incapable one. It was frustrating to be unable to keep up with the group and perform like everyone else.

A huge difference between those early families and the families of today is that the early ones knew the power and importance of good food, and we do not. They knew which foods were needed to create and maintain superior health, and they knew where and how to get that food regardless of the terrain they lived in. Much of this wisdom has been lost over the past several hundred years with the rise of the Industrial Revolution.

By the time the 17th century had come and gone, machinery and other laborsaving devices were proliferating rapidly across Europe, luring us away from the soil. Perhaps we were attracted by the endless amount of work the machines could do, by their tirelessness, or the sheer power they exhibited. Maybe we were bored after thousands of years of plowing and planting. Whatever it was, we were fascinated with things that tick and click or whirr and pound. Because of this, machine culture began to flourish side-by-side with agriculture, and the idea of an easier life was probably as mesmerizing as it was naïve.

Early pilgrims who came to America were looking for spiritual freedom – but the rich, fertile soil they found was a nice bonus. Perhaps it never occurred to them that the famines following crop failures and the miserable health conditions in European cities were deeply connected to the decline of soils and falling levels of nutrition in the foods that were available there.

Neither has it occurred to anyone today that America's Founding Fathers were able to imagine a place like America, then come up with the strength and energy to build such a place because they were eating food grown in the living soil that was everywhere here, at least in the beginning. Today, we barely have enough energy to change jobs let alone envision, start, and win a revolution.

The Real Costs of Poor Health

If you don't want to bother learning to feed yourself differently, then you don't really want to heal yourself. Expecting someone to give you a pill or cut out your parts and make you magically better is childish, irresponsible, and doesn't get to the source of your problem. This kind of expectation is like demanding that others do for you what you are unwilling to do for yourself. The medical doctors I know well would love to have patients who would take responsibility for doing those things that will enhance the body's efforts to heal itself *and* who are realistic about what the M.D. can offer. To start a true healing process, it's almost a given that you will have to change your diet to real, whole, organic food.

If you think you cannot afford whole, high-nutrition, organic foods, get out a piece of paper and pencil and add up the monthly cost of the following items:

What you spend on groceries each month _____

Eating out: breakfast, lunches, and dinners _____

The cost of your medical insurance _____

The cost of your dental insurance _____

Orthodontic work for you and your children _____

The cost of your vision insurance _____

Glasses, contact lenses, lens cleaning supplies _____

Co-pay amounts not covered by insurance _____

The cost of specialists you must see _____

Alternative health practitioners you visit _____

Prescription medicines & drugs you must buy _____

Over-the-counter cold and flu medicines _____

Over-the-counter arthritis medicines _____

Over-the-counter allergy medicines _____

Over the counter asthma medicines _____

Over-the-counter digestive upset medicines _____

Psychological counseling _____

Special education/tutoring for ADHD children _____

Sick days off – due to fatigue or illness _____

Vitamins and minerals you buy _____

Herbal supplements you buy _____

The cost of enzymes and digestive aids _____

Aspirin, dry skin lotions, toothpaste, deodorants, and make-up to cover up your headaches, bad skin, bad breath, and poor body odor _____

The cost of poor productivity that results from irritability and tension in family relationships _____

The cost of nursing home services for your elderly parents _____

The cost of special shoes, clothing, chairs, canes, braces, walkers, beds, stairs, showers, toilets, etc. _____

The cost of special diets for allergies, illness, weight loss, etc. _____

The cost/membership fees of weight loss centers or groups _____

The cost of extra clothing that must be maintained as weight goes up and down _____

The cost of physical therapy programs _____

The cost of gyms, aerobic programs, or exercise programs to lose weight _____

The cost of gasoline to get to doctors, clinics, gyms, and therapies of any kind _____

The cost of hotel and motel rooms or alternative sleeping arrangements for family during hospital care _____

The cost of days lost at work so you could
stay home and take care of a sick family
member   _____

TOTAL COST OF POOR HEALTH   _____

Now, take a really good look at these costs and the total. This should do several things. First, it should give you a fair idea of what you could really afford to spend on *good* food.

Second, it should make you see the amount of time, energy, and money you spend compensating for mediocre-to-poor health. We could carry the argument for high nutrition food even further by adding in the costs of a job that you take just so you can have medical benefits that you know you need because of poor health. In that case, you could legitimately add the cost of special work clothes, a car to drive to the job, gasoline, mileage, insurance, the need to hire someone to clean, cook, or cut the grass because you no longer have time, the cost of child care, the potential increase in food costs because of a greater reliance on convenience foods, and anything else associated with the job.

Third, ask yourself, "To what degree do the costs and activities in this list seem normal?" The more normal they seem, the more caught you are in the thinking produced by our current food system. What could you be doing with that same time, energy, and money if you were perfectly healthy and free to do whatever you wanted? Would you read more...tinker in your workshop...take swimming lessons...make love...sew, knit, quilt, or crochet more...invent things...go hiking...have a child...build something...take a trip to a place you've always wanted to visit...write a book...go dancing...cook gourmet meals...grow roses...visit antique shops...sit in the back yard and enjoy a peaceful afternoon...attend the theater or a rodeo...see a live basketball game...join a yoga or meditation group...work one job instead of two...allow one spouse to quit work and stay home?

Lastly, can you even imagine being supremely healthy – or would this leave you feeling left out of the circle of family, friends, and coworkers who are struggling with illness, fatigue, the effects of degeneration, and catastrophic disease? What would you talk about if you didn't have your own complaints and physical difficulties to add to the general conversation that goes on around you every day?

The important lesson in all of this is: don't tell yourself that you can't afford good, whole, high-nutrition food because I'm going to turn that around and tell you emphatically that you can't afford *not* to buy good food! If you can't afford to buy it, then grow it.

It is the absence of this kind of food that leads to illness or disease in the first place. Bacteria and viruses are not at fault; they are important members of the physical family with the job of breaking down old carbon-based matter and recycling it for further use. When there is a fall-off of high level immune function, our cells devolve into lower forms of expression that we call bacteria or viruses, and we appear to have a disease with specific symptoms. Bacteria is the *result* of disease, not the cause of it. [34]

Your genes are not at fault. Genes are triggered into action – or fail to be triggered into action – by the subtle frequency waves given off by molecules of vitamins, minerals, and enzymes in your food. Those who blame our genes for illness are akin to those who blame rape victims for being raped. Genes are not the problem. Genes that do not work properly are the result of poor nutrition.

This is not to say that those doing research into our genes are misguided or wasting their time, for there is much to be learned; and if you step back far enough to get a bigger picture, you will see a definite civilizational goal among human beings to recognize and understand the hidden details of life and creation.

We are extremely creative beings searching for new and exciting yet practical applications of the Source Energy from which we all come. We know there is a Source. That is not in question. But what are the possibilities of that Source? What can we become? Who knows what we can learn to do, to correct, to create and re-create if we understand the fine points of what makes us tick? I love science, I love the physical world we live in. I love the *meta*-physical worlds of spirit and energy, and I love having a creative life myself. My concern at this point is that we may not survive as a group to continue exploring and creating if we do not correct the way we feed ourselves.

❖

---

[34] Christopher Bird, *The Persecution and Trial of Gaston Naessens* (Tiburon, CA: HJ Kramer Inc, 1991) p. 4-11.

Chemical Agriculture is Born

In the same way that Weston Price and his peers were struggling with the deluge of degenerative diseases that appeared in humans between 1900 and 1950, difficultties in animal breeding and crop production caught the attention of veterinarians and agricultural scientists. Animals were also suffering from a host of degenerative diseases, while plants were being attacked by insects and fungus everywhere.

A few men, like Dr. Charles Northern and William Albrecht, Professor of Agronomy at the University of Missouri, had been seriously encouraging farmers to put great effort into re-mineralizing and restoring soils, but by the mid 1950s they were working against the rising tide of big business and the chemical corporations that had entered the world of agriculture after World War II.

During the war, a number of chemical engineering companies had produced and stockpiled tons of chemicals for making bombs. When the war ended, they were left with no markets for these chemicals. Then they discovered agriculture. People were leaving farms and moving to the cities, looking for jobs and big money. As farm families fractured, there were not enough hands to do the work. With falling crop production, increasing pressure from pests and diseases, rising numbers of people in the world who expected someone else to grow the food they needed, and an American self-image as a sort of "food savior" to the world, agriculture was ripe for an influx of chemicals.

Within a very short time, chemical companies were using the stockpiled bomb chemicals to make NPK fertilizers. Use of these fertilizers caused further imbalances in soils and plants, which then necessitated pesticides, herbicides, and finally fungicides. Soon these chemicals were being developed by the thousands. Chemical salesmen went out across the country, peddling these potions to farmers and convincing the agriculture departments of many universities that they needed to recommend the chemical concoctions to the farmers in the area. When department heads showed resistance, large sums of money were given to the university to "help" with research that would prove the usefulness of the chemicals.

Before long, a whole new generation of young farmers – all university trained – began using chemicals for everything from plant growth to insect, weed, and disease control. The traditional wisdom of constantly restoring the soil was abandoned as old-fashioned.

Once NPK fertilizers were in widespread use, farmers no longer needed animals for the rich manure that had been composted and applied to soils. The animals were sold off. Once the animals were gone, the animal barns were no longer needed and fell into disrepair.

The new, young farmers bought big tractors and big equipment, plowed under the pastures, orchards, and gardens once used to grow a variety of healthy feeds for cows, horses, and chickens, then planted everything to a single crop. The farm, once a closely related community of plants, animals, and people that was self-sufficient and self-maintaining, began to disintegrate. Instead of tending a lot of little crops whose incomes and losses served to balance each other over the course of a year and prevent a catastrophic loss, the farmer now went into high-risk debt, gambling that he could make enough money from a single crop large enough to sell in the world export markets. However, once into the export markets, he lost control of what he could charge. Instead of going up, the farmer's income dropped, and now he had huge debts whose payments had to be deferred "until harvest."

Trying to make a few more dollars, he sold every ounce of grain he had produced, failing to hold enough seed in reserve for the next year. It was easy to believe the chemical salesman's claim that he could purchase better seed the following year, seed that would supposedly germinate faster, resist more diseases, produce a bigger crop, and make him more money.

Instead, caught up in corporate-style agriculture, many farmers couldn't make the payments and lost the entire farm, which was then bought up by corporate-style managers who were not interested in restoring soils, and who knew little or nothing about raising high-nutrition foods. They were interested in getting a crop to market in the cheapest, quickest manner possible and getting paid.

Today, many farmers use chemicals and poisons because they don't know how to raise food any other way. They are doing what *their* fathers did, and since their fathers were the early chemical farmers, that's all they know. The old ways of maintaining healthy livestock in order to continuously restore the soil have been lost. Many farmers no longer know how to take care of animals, barns are expensive to build, physical labor is no longer fashionable, and families no longer live and work together.

Specialization has become the way of most farming today. Some raise beef or hogs, some raise wheat, some raise fruit, others raise cabbage, or chickens. As farming fractured into hundreds of specialty practices, it became more and more difficult to see the whole picture.

When a single farmer is raising corn, beef, chickens, fruit, and everything else he eats and needs, he isn't interested in doing something that will be bad for one part of his operation even if he thinks it would be good for another part of the operation.

When you can't see the whole, it's easy to let go of the little practices that maintain balance. They no longer seem important or necessary or related to what you're doing. Today, we have a situation in which it's every man for himself, and the wheat farmer doesn't care what the beef farmer needs, nor does the beef or pork farmer pay attention to what the chicken or the fruit farmer needs. And none of them seem to know or understand what the human being needs.

Real farming has long been one of the most demanding professions there is. Among other things, it requires you to be a scientist, keenly observant naturalist, animal breeder, weatherman, veterinarian, animal mid-wife, plant breeder, machine operator, machine repairman, carpenter, bookkeeper, manager, entrepreneur, and physical laborer, as well as your own source of self-discipline, motivation, and ongoing self-education. Few people are interested in farming to begin with, and when they discover how many diverse skills and talents are required, they go elsewhere looking for easier jobs.

Today, foods and farming have gotten caught up in the mass-market mindset of industrial production and competition. Foods are now handled in ways similar to clothing and fashion design. Every year new "food concepts" are carefully created, designed, packaged, and presented at big conventions attended by salesmen who buy for the big grocery store chains, mini-marts, gas station chains, and small independent stores. The hope is always that something in this year's line-up will be a hit, become a fad, and then move into the category where it is thought of as a staple in American kitchens. The problem is that these new foods are not really foods. They contain a few skeletalized or chemicalized remains of what might have been food at one time, mixed up with sugar, food coloring, and artificial flavoring agents. They have pretty boxes or wrappers presenting pictures that look like food, and sometimes they smell like food. You can eat them as if they are food, but they aren't *real* food capable of rebuilding and restoring bodies. They are pretend foods used to make money in the annual money-making competitions of the industrial markets.

Competition implies a lack of caring for the other guy. When we stop caring for others, society shatters. When the goal is to make money, that's one thing. When the goal is to feed yourself, that's another thing. And when the aim is to feed yourself in ways that sustain you in excellent health, that's something else altogether.

A Little Food Education

I grew up in the thumb area of Michigan in a large family. My grandmother lived to be 100 years old, and her father – my great-grandfather – lived to 101 years old. Grandma gave birth to 14 healthy children, raised them all, and until she was in her mid-80s, she continued to live on her farm and raise or grow her own food. She took chicken, beef, butter, milk, and vegetables to her friends in town who were 20 years younger and already confined to beds or wheelchairs with poor health, giving them "heck for thinking they were old and useless." When she left the farm, she traveled the world for some years, then settled down in her house in town, where she stayed until her mid-90s.

For a long time, I expected that my parents and I would live to be very old, just like my grandparents and great-grandparents. Then my father discovered he had cancer. He survived that, but died at the age of 69 from congestive heart failure, a complicating factor of emphysema. I was already suffering from rheumatoid arthritis before he died. My husband was suffering from severe asthma and had long ago been diagnosed with chronic obstructive pulmonary disease. For five years, he was barely able to drag himself to work during the winter because it was almost impossible for him to breathe in cold weather.

My husband and I were in our mid-40s at that time, and it was clear that at our present rate of deterioration, we might not make it any further than my father. I looked at the extraordinary good health of my immediate ancestors and felt I had to begin learning how to heal myself. What I have learned came too late to help my father, but it was not too late to help myself or my husband, the rest of the family, and many others as well.

When I ask people who attend my classes what they know about food in general, the answers they give are excellent examples of the extreme confusion that most people have about food today. "Meat is taboo, especially red meat...and vegetarianism is in...soy is good...fat is the culprit in heart disease...milk is the cause of all kinds of sinus problems, allergies, mucus, and ear-nose-and-throat infections...eggs, cheese, and fat are the source of both high cholesterol and heart problems...whereas milk, wheat, beans, and peanuts cause life-threatening allergies or gastrointestinal upsets."

When I started studying nutrition and came across the work of Weston Price, I stacked my grandmother's good health and life-long diet on top of Price's information and asked myself, "How is it that our ancestors were as healthy as they were when they ate all kinds of meat, fat, milk, cheese, eggs, and grains without cancers, heart disease, allergies, high cholesterol, and numerous forms of food intolerance?"

I had been mostly vegetarian and had not been drinking milk for over ten years at the time I came down with rheumatoid arthritis. I was also keeping up with all the latest articles on what we should be eating and was diligently applying these guidelines to my life. But observations of my grandmother's life and the things I was learning about real nutrition were lining up in direct opposition to what was being printed in popular magazines. Real food seemed to be a complete contradiction to what was advertised on television or announced on the boxes and labels of the many foods I purchased.

If you are getting your education about food from the magazines that fill grocery store shelves, you will end up going in circles and not knowing what to eat and what to avoid. Someone says eat lots of this, and someone else says eat lots of that, while someone new contradicts both of them. If you are basing your decision of what to eat on the information circulating in the popular culture, you are going to end up in a physically degenerated condition because no one is writing or talking about real food or the fact that there is not enough nutrition in the food that's out there. Everyone is grasping at straws.

To make matters worse, researchers are hired by companies to "validate" certain products and are paid handsomely to come to specific conclusions that help marketing and advertising departments sell the new foods by creating false beliefs.

In some cases, early researchers drew erroneous conclusions that did not hold up over time. A good many doctors, as well as scientists and researchers, looking through the original research of their peers barely glanced at the methodology and numbers. They read only the summary conclusions at the end of the research, adopting these conclusions without ever evaluating the actual research methodology and numbers, thus spreading the misinformation. Everyone was assuming that others had read and carefully evaluated the actual research, which was not the case. [35]

People writing for magazines were also not reading the original research that had been done in various studies; they were only reading what other popular press writers had written. Thus, everyone was perpetuating the circle of misinformation until it became entrenched as dogma, and food processing industries grew up based on the demands of people who had been supplied with serious misinformation.

I ran into this dilemma when I decided to try writing articles for the popular press. Pieces that focused on what I had learned about food and health were quickly rejected. Finally, I was told by one editor, who wanted to use part of one article and cut out all the relevant pieces, that they did not want to print something that would make their advertisers look bad, and that every health magazine had doctors, nutritionists, and advisors on their boards who were vested in the present system.

❖

There is no more destructive idea in the culture today than the idea that you can live, thrive, and stay healthy on "manufactured" foods. You may get by for a while, you may survive for a time eating foods that are empty of nutrition, but you will not feel well during that survival, you will not perform well, and you will not last very long before something in the body/mind system gives out. Certainly, the last thing you want to do is trigger your family weak spot. For some families the weak spot is multiple sclerosis, for some it is high blood pressure, cancer, or a weak heart. In others, it is schizophrenia or manic-depressive disorder, perhaps a tendency toward weak lungs or kidney disease.

Once you trigger the illness that runs in your family, it is not a simple case of eating better, taking a few vitamins or herbs, and expecting to recover. You must literally embark on a total rebuilding program in which you constantly supply yourself with top-quality nutrition at a rate of about four times the normal rates until all the poorly built cells that were constructed under the old nutritional program have died off and been replaced by new, healthy ones. My own personal experience has been that a big improvement can be made in one year, but if you stick with it for three to five years, you will end up rebuilding your

---

[35] Sally Fallon, *The Oiling of America*, a lecture given in 1998.

entire body/mind system to the point that some people may not recognize you.

You are not destined to be sick, ill, or suffer from degenerative disease. If you give the body what it needs to constantly repair and rebuild itself, then good health is the normal state of affairs, healing is a natural process, and high energy and longevity are the results. Your body knows how to heal itself. You just need to know how to support its efforts to do so. Good food is the foundation of any healing program.

Presently, there is mass-produced, factory food, and there is *real* food. Real food has been taking a bashing, and a great deal of misunderstanding has been circulating in this country for years. Real foods seldom cause diseases and allergies. After all, we thrived on these foods for 10,000 years and are supremely adapted to them.

For example, lots of people in this country will tell you they are allergic to wheat. But what they are eating is not really wheat. It is a highly over-processed, skeletonized, bleached-out version of what was once whole wheat. Almost all of the vitamins, minerals, amino acids, natural oils, subtle metabolic co-factors, and digestive enzymes have been removed. The result is a useless substance that irritates the body, thus, the apparent "allergy to wheat." It is the same story with many other foods.

Real food is whole and full of living enzymes. Science has never been able to synthesize enzymes because it has never learned to synthesize life.

Living food is full of organic vitamins and minerals. The key word here is *organic*. Lots of manufacturers are fully aware that food processing strips food of important nutrients, so they add a few vitamins and minerals back in to the foods they process. But the vitamins and minerals that a manufacturer puts into a food item are *inorganic* and not at all the same as the vitamins and minerals that the processing took out.

When a food plant such as a green bean produces sulfur (a mineral) or a cantaloupe produces retinol (vitamin A), these minerals and vitamins are *organic*, which means they are sized, shaped, and ready for use in a living body. They also have additional subtle co-factors and wave energies in them that work synergistically with all of the other nutrient factors in that food. The body welcomes these food nutrients immediately and uses them easily. Our ancestors lived to advanced ages in a healthy condition on all kinds of meats, fats, milks, cheeses, eggs, grains, and small amounts of vegetables and fruits.

However, the body has a great deal of difficulty utilizing inorganic minerals and chemically synthesized vitamins because these molecules are too big or are oddly shaped, or they do not have the subtle energies that produce the dozens of secondary effects which help coordinate the full power of the metabolic reaction the body is trying to organize and carry out. A good analogy here might be the difference between trying to build a fire with dry, seasoned wood, and trying to build a fire with wet wood. The wood is still wood whether wet or dry, and it will burn eventually, but in the meantime the warming effect of the fire is greatly reduced. You may have to use a lot of paper, cardboard, or kindling to keep it going, and there is a lot of smoke that clouds the air, as well as creosote that clogs the chimney with unused combustible products.

The body *will* try to use artificial foods with their inorganic minerals and synthetic vitamins – not to mention the food coloring, chemical preservatives, flavoring agents, pesticide residues, and heavy metals, but the results are less than optimum and there are a lot of wastes and lost energy that clutter up the system.

A few people in my classes have tried to insist that our ancestors did not live to advanced ages in a healthy condition. They have tried to tell me that life expectancy has never been higher than it is today here in the U.S. and a few other First World countries. They have tried to get me to accept the idea that our ancestors were ignorant primitives that lived to the age of 35 then died miserably. The truth is that there *have* been periods of time when we died too soon and periods of time when we have lived to ripe old ages. When the Industrial Revolution began, we set forces in motion that played havoc with our health. But those who stayed on the farms or close to the land did not suffer the poor health of those in the cities.

If you have been narrowly educated in public schools and believe that the only history that counts is the Western white man's version…if you think that First World countries have the best way of life and Third World people are ignorant savages…if you believe that you know more and know better (rather than knowing *differently*) than those who came before you….if you are looking only at the last few hundred years of the Western white man's history…then learning more and more about real food will probably cause some serious perceptual upsets.

As our European ancestors were coaxed off their land to work in the first factories, the need arose to provide them with food. As people began moving into cities to be near the factories of the Industrial

Revolution, their diets suffered and so did their immune systems. As the Industrial Revolution spread, physical, mental, emotional, and spiritual health plummeted along with longevity.

Gone was the high resistance to disease and infections. Bubonic plague, known as the Black Death, accompanied this transition from country to city, from good food to poor food, sweeping across Europe and wiping out half of the population. Many died early, miserable deaths from measles, smallpox, cholera, tuberculosis, and pneumonia. We have been trying to recover our health security ever since.

People like to say we are living longer than we were two or three hundred years ago because it makes them feel better. But before the Industrial Revolution, before the days of big machinery, large cities, and gigantic factories, those who evolved stable cultures, good food supplies, and cooperative societies tended to live very long, useful lives, healthy and alert to the end. It was a frequently observed fact that old European women who emigrated to America in the early 1900s, but kept their former ways of raising food, cooking, and eating, often ended up healthy and strong to the age of 100 or more while they nursed and then buried their much younger daughters who had adopted the white-flour/white-sugar diet of the New World.

Somewhere along the line, in an effort to keep food flowing into the cities, Europeans began adopting a diet of white flour, white sugar, canned vegetables, jams and jellies, alcohol, and sweets. Perhaps remnants of such a diet survived from Rome to blossom once more in the courts of Marseilles and London. And who knows where Rome may have gotten such haute cuisine, maybe from Egypt or even Babylon? Diets live and die along with the people who adopt them as eating habits.

European missionaries carried the white man's diet around the world with them, becoming a potent wedge between people and the healing lifestyles they had evolved over thousands of years. Everywhere they went, disruption of indigenous lives followed. People who lived in close relationship to the land, who loved the land, who depended on the continuation of their feeding traditions for maintenance of their high immunity, were suddenly forced out of their sustaining routines, into schools and churches, and onto barren soils. They were fed Western foods right along with Western religion. The result was confusion, disease, psychological malaise, and death everywhere the missionaries went.

Today we do not have missionaries to contend with, we have marketing departments. A great deal of misinformation has been generated by over-enthusiastic marketing programs designed to get sales moving for a product that just isn't selling. Once the misinformation gets out there, we build on it, creating a labyrinth of wrong turns in terms of our diet. If we do not correct this, we simply will not survive. ❖

8
Real Food

AS I WRITE these words I am 62-years-old, which is still on the young side in my view! I do not take any kind of medication, I have recovered from arthritis, and I work 12 to 16 hours a day, seven days a week, doing a wide range of physical, mental, emotional, and spiritual work.

Here at the farm I eat a base diet of whole, organic foods that I have grown or raised myself, take supplements as needed, follow regular detox routines as a form of healing and maintenance, and exercise as part of the daily work routine. Yet, I am not a purist in what I do here. Some days have no exercise. Some months are too busy for detox procedures. Some days include cake or cookies, potato chips and salsa, perhaps wine or beer, and I have not been willing to give up ice cream entirely. Yet, the mainstay of my base diet is so nutritious that I do quite well with an occasional excursion into the world of goodies and junk food.

I have come to expect that I will have prodigious amounts of energy, that I will feel good a majority of the time, and that colds, flu, or other illness and disease will pass by without affecting me. When I do eat foods from "the outside," I can tell by the immediate dip in my energy and mood that I have eaten empty food. If I keep it up too long, I may have a blunt reminder of the weak point in my physical system. Perhaps, I might do even better for much longer in life if I was more purist in my eating, but humans do not live by bread alone.

I have family, friends, and visitors that do not understand why I work as long and hard as I do to produce my own food. Many have asked me why I don't just take it easy and go to the store. I have several reasons for growing my own.

First, I learned from an old chiropractor who was a great healer, "Sometimes the easy way is not so easy after a while." The grocery store may be easy when you're young, have money, and are healthy. But if you continue to eat manufactured foods without nutrition, you will age quickly, suffer serious degeneration, and soon life is not so easy any more.

Second, I want *real* food, the tried-and-true kind that our ancestors depended on, and you can't get that from the junk-food or even the grocery store. Real food is food that comes straight from the garden, the field, or the animal without a lot of processing.

Third, vegetables and fruits grow in the soil where many kinds of bacteria live, including staph and strep. Since plants must defend themselves against these bacteria much like we have to, they produce factors called *pacifarins* as their protective defense. When we eat the food grown locally and in our own gardens, these pacifarins are passed on to us and help protect us against the forms of staph, strep, and other antagonistic bacteria that exist in our local environment. Since each locality has unique genetic variations of bacteria, there is a bit of added protection and support that comes to us through the foods that grow in that location.

Fourth, real food that is whole and unprocessed contains factors called *auxones*. These are factors grown by Mother Nature that help you digest and absorb the specific vitamins and co-vitamins that are contained in any given kind of food. In other words, foods that contain Vitamin A will have auxones that help you absorb and utilize that vitamin in the body. Foods with lots of Vitamin D will have auxones that help your body take in that vitamin. The same is true of the other vitamins and minerals found in whole, unprocessed food.

For these reasons, I grow as much of my own food as possible. I raise pasture-fed beef; drink whole, unpasteurized milk and cream; churn my own butter; make my own yogurt and a few cheeses. I buy organic wheat directly from a farmer in North Dakota, grind the wheat and bake my own breads, muffins, and rolls before the natural oils in the flour turn rancid. My daughter and I raise our own chickens and enjoy their eggs regularly. In my garden, you will find corn, broccoli, peas, potatoes, tomatoes, celery, cabbage, cauliflower, Brussels sprouts, kohlrabi, radishes, onions, turnips, carrots, beans, beets, cucumbers, summer squash, butternut squash, pumpkins, zucchini, okra, ten different kinds of lettuce, cantaloupe, honeydew melon, watermelon, strawberries, and raspberries. I make my own catsup, vinegars, jams, jellies, pickles, and juice. I also grow almost two dozen culinary herbs, and collect a dozen other medicinal herbs that grow wild on our property.

What I don't or can't grow here – like grapefruit, spelt, or lemons – I try to buy directly from other farmers across the U.S. who know the value and power of real food and who make an effort to grow the highest quality food they can.

I don't always choose organic food. Instead, I look for high-nutrition food. You can tell quite a bit by the size, color, smell, and texture whether the nutrition is decent. When something has been picked too early, it will never develop the natural sugars and high-level nutrition it should have. A good indication of nutrition level is how heavy the food is. A bushel of top quality, nutrient-dense wheat weighs 62 lbs. A bushel of deficient, low nutrition wheat weighs 60 lbs; what seems like a minor difference makes all the difference in the world.

Another good indication of nutrition level is how much natural sweetness the fruit or vegetable has. How sweet something is can often be assessed by smell and sometimes by its outside color and texture.

Knowing the natural size of produce is also helpful. Finding a gigantic peach on the grocery store shelf may impress you, but it may be just a bloated, dry, tough, and tasteless mass. If it doesn't have good color and you can't smell its perfume, it will probably be a very disappointing peach. If you paid a premium price because of its size, you have allowed yourself to be cheated.

Once in awhile, I get something at the grocery store that proves to be very low in quality once I get it home. Examples might be oranges or lemons that are almost completely dried up inside when I cut them open or a cucumber that turns moldy the day after purchase. If this is the case, I take it back and ask for my money back. Most people don't think you can do this with food, but you can. And the message it sends to the buyer at the store is: "Don't try to sell me garbage. I'm not settling for that. Find better produce."

Really good stores go out of their way to find the things their customers love. If they are going to do this, however, they need to know what you like. Tell them! Communication is essential. If grocery stores are going to become suppliers of real food, they need to hear from you. When they respond to your requests, thank them.

When people discover that our food supply has almost no nutrition in it, they often feel angry, outraged, confused, or helpless. They begin blaming the government and various organizations for trapping them in an economy that does not value or understand the soil, agriculture, or the importance of high-nutrition food. They feel they're on a conveyor belt that will deliver them to the realms of poor and degenerating health where they will then be trapped by the pharmaceutical companies who demand outrageous prices for the drugs that will keep them alive. This attitude is not really helpful unless you consider the fact that anger is really "change energy" – the way we feel when we want something to change right now!

What is helpful is to realize that the government is run by a lot of people who are just like you and me. They're trying to do their best, they don't want anyone to get sick from eating something "bad," and many actually believe that the best way to prevent this is to process the heck out of the food substance until there's absolutely nothing left in it that might cause a bad reaction in anyone. Unfortunately, there is then nothing left in the food in terms of nutrition – and the plan to make our food supply safer is now backfiring. People have degenerated so dramatically that immune systems are extremely fragile and can no longer handle irritants of any sort. By removing all the factors that might cause a reaction—the vitamins, minerals, fats, oils, and enzymes—the food becomes tasteless, colorless, and lacks texture. To restore the taste, color and texture, food processors add artificial vitamins, inorganic minerals, chemical colors and texturizers, white sugar to sweeten, and sometimes vegetable fats in the form of polyunsaturated oils. Since the body has no use for these, it simply does the best it can, but over time, the result is disaster.

A couple of years ago, I was teaching a class in *Getting Well Again, Naturally,* and a young woman in her late-20s was attending. For years, she had slowly begun avoiding one real food group after the next because everything she read in the popular press talked about how each was bad for you in one way or another. Now, she was having trouble with her menstrual periods, headaches, irritation, depression, fatigue, constipation, and difficulty with concentration and focus.

As we talked about real food, about meats, milk, eggs, and cheese, about fats and cholesterol, grains, beans, nuts, vegetables, and fruits, she began to grasp the truth about real food.

At lunch, we were all talking when I noticed her sitting in her chair, ignoring her food and staring off into the distance for some time.

"Are you all right?" I asked her, wondering if she was ill or somehow uncomfortable.

"My god..." she exclaimed, "...the vastness of the illusion..."

I knew instantly that she was seeing through the illusions that had grown up around food. All at once, the widespread ignorance about real food and the continuous marketing campaigns that push artificial, manufactured foods at us from every direction were clear and in perspective for her.

If you truly want to heal, one of the most important steps you can take is to return to real food. ❖

9
Meat

WHEN I FIRST STARTED to raise cows and chickens, it was because I wanted the manure for my vegetable garden. As was typical for those who have lost their connection to the soil and the food chain, it never occurred to me to think of these animals as food at first. When I ended up with 13 roosters in the first batch of chickens, and the cow I bought gave birth to a calf only three days after I brought her home, an old-time farmer across the road suggested I think about raising my own beef and chicken. I shied away from the idea for a while, but finally, with considerable trepidation, decided to learn how to kill and dress my own meat. I prepared long and deeply for the day, my tears falling freely. Yet nothing prepared me for the extraordinary differences between this meat and the meat I had purchased at the grocery store.

What I had raised with great love produced such tender, tasty, melt-in-your-mouth meat that I could hardly believe the difference. I hadn't done anything exotic or unusual with my animals. I just made sure there was plenty of pasture to run in, good grass and grazing for both cows and chickens, freedom to mingle, a few grains, and supplements to keep them healthy. I also refused to use hormones or antibiotics.

Asking an animal to give the gift of its life so that I could eat was a powerfully humbling experience that deepened my awareness of the value of life and made me acutely conscious of my interdependence with all things. It taught me to make sure that my animals had a good life while they were alive and to honor them and their needs because in the end, filling their needs filled mine. I have learned much.

The chickens run around their 1½ acre yard freely, scratching up crawling bugs, chasing flying insects (bugs and insects are high-protein foods), eating grasses and weeds (grasses and weeds are really herbal foods), and watching out for predators such as raccoons and chicken hawks. They come and go from the chicken coop, rest in the shade of the big hickory tree, mate freely, and defend their place in the pecking order with gusto. Every day I replenish their grains (usually corn, oats, and wheat) and water, sprinkling a little montmorillonite clay in both food and water to prevent salmonella in their wonderful eggs, which have bright, fluorescent-orange yolks.

When it is time to cull the flock, I kill them as quickly and cleanly as possible. With great care, I remove the oil sack back by the tail, then the intestines, being careful not to break them open for this would release bacteria and e-coli into the cavity of the bird. Then I scrub and rinse them, putting them into the freezer or the stockpot immediately.

In contrast, chickens raised in a commercial operation often spend a very short, miserable life in a wire cage that is roughly 5" x 8". They can't even turn around let alone run around. They eat synthetic feeds with low quality synthetic proteins in them. Their feed is supplemented with estrogen-based hormones to plump up their breast for market and antibiotics to keep them alive long enough to get to market. Their manure is carried off by one conveyor, and their pale, tasteless eggs are carried off by another. Often they are riddled with disease and cancers by the time they are sent to the food processor.

The processors kill the sick, stressed birds and put the carcass on a moving assembly line. There, a mechanical reamer will ream out the intestines, breaking them open and spreading bacteria all over the inside cavity of the bird. The processors think that any bacteria will be taken care of by rinsing the carcass in antibacterial solutions and irradiating the meat. But sometimes the antibacterial rinses kill only the most susceptible bacteria, leaving the more persistent and deadly to flourish and grow, and irradiation is very destructive to humans who eat the meat.

The meat itself is tough, rubbery, and tasteless. Besides the absence of nutrition, there are residues of whatever chemicals, heavy metals, antibiotics, and hormones the chicken ingested. The result is difficulty for us in digesting it. Food sensitivities and allergies appear in us; not because of the meat, but because our bodies do not like the chemicals or heavy metals in the meat. As for the estrogen-based hormones used to make chicken breasts nice and plump, I suspect that the white meat fad that spread across the country over the past decade has added more than a little pressure to the wave of estrogen-based breast cancers that have been appearing in record numbers of women across the country, not to mention the early maturation of many young girls.

When you buy meat today you are never sure what you are going to get. But the chances are quite good that you will be buying something that was raised in a feedlot or cage and whose nutritional deficiencies were severe. Any animal raised in a nutritionally deficient environment is going to be nutritionally deficient food and will unbalance your own health and physical system.

Cows, and pigs as well, do very well living in the open on good grasses and pasture that has a wide spectrum of weeds (herbs) in it so they can doctor themselves by going after what their system needs. And they do a great job of this!

If you buy beef that shrinks by a third when you cook it, you have purchased meat from a cow that got too little calcium and too much potassium. Many farmers keep their cows in feedlots and buy feed that was fertilized with NPK fertilizers. Since calcium is so easily chemically-bound by other mineral factors when the soil is out of balance, newly growing grain will uptake potassium from the N-P-K in the soil, using it as a substitute for calcium.

When the cow eats this kind of grain, it gets heavy doses of potassium instead of the necessary calcium. This is especially true if the cow is already deficient in magnesium, selenium, and boron. For the cow, the result of too much potassium is a lush, watery, bloated body that looks like a solid weight gain. It makes the cow look big and healthy. This is a dangerous illusion because the cow is actually much more disease-prone than normal and very susceptible to insects and pathogens, which is why antibiotics and other drugs are routinely administered.

In the old days, before we started trying to rush the process, farmers raised cows on pasture grass, vegetables, hay, and plenty of mineral salts. This way of feeding created meat with great flavor and texture.

After slaughter and dressing, the sides of beef were allowed to hang in the cooler for two or three, even four, weeks. During this time, living enzymes (mainly cathepsin) in the muscle and tissue of the beef would go to work breaking down the tough muscle fibers. The longer these enzymes were allowed to work, the more tender the beef would become. The goal was to allow the enzymes to do a good job of breaking down fiber and tenderizing without allowing total disintegration of the meat. By the third week, someone would have to go into the cooler or ice house every day and wipe off the thin layer of fine bluish-white mold on the outside of the carcass. This simple care step prevented the meat from going bad while it tenderized. When the process was complete, the meat was melt-in-your-mouth tender, had retained the rich flavor of grass-fed beef, and was ready for your body to digest without undue exhaustion of digestive juices or enzymes.

Nowadays, cows are kept in small pens and feedlots where we try to fatten them quickly with corn and other grains. Cows that eat grain suffer from acid stomach, which upsets their digestion in the same way it disrupts ours. This also interferes with mineral absorption, and thus, the meat lacks texture and flavor. When the corn is potassium-laden instead of rich in calcium, their tissues swell with water.

When the cow appears to have gained enough weight, it is sent off to market where it is killed and then hung in a cooler for perhaps only a week before carving. During this period, the hanging beef loses quite a bit of water through evaporation. Meat packing companies won't let the meat hang long enough to really tenderize because it loses too much weight through this evaporation of water from tissues. Every pound of water loss cuts down the financial profit because beef is sold by the pound. Thus, ready or not, it is cut, wrapped, and sent off to market. When you buy it and cook it, the rest of the water evaporates, the meat shrinks, and what remains in the pan is tough, leathery, and tasteless. It is also difficult to chew, difficult to digest, and without the payload of nutrition that it should have had.

❖

In a human population, the shortage of calcium and an excess of potassium in our grains and meat has the same effect on us as it does on a cow. We get heavy and bloated-looking. That swollen, bloated look is one of the first signs of malnutrition, the later signs being a severely swollen belly while the rest of the body looks like a skeleton. At present, the entire U.S. population is swollen, bloated-looking, and bears considerable resemblance to the proverbial Pillsbury doughboy.[36] The

---

[36] *Pillsbury* is a registered trademark of the Pillsbury Corporation.

result is that we think we need to go on a diet. As soon as we start dieting, we get even less of the nutrition our body needs, and the downward degenerative spiral continues. The real truth is that we need high-nutrition food.

Long ago, it was a tradition that when a cow was killed and dressed, almost every part of it was used for something. People ate the muscle meats along with the glands, the organs, the brain, and other parts. The hides were tanned to make leather, the hooves, tail, and bones were scrubbed and put into stockpots to make gelatin-rich, mineral-rich beef stock, and the fat was rendered into tallow.

Some of these parts, especially the glands, had to be used right away, and as the grocery store system grew, buyers hesitated to buy anything that wouldn't keep for at least a week or two. Gradually, people shopping for their food in grocery stores forgot about the old ways of eating. They tended to be mesmerized by the thick, red steaks and roasts from the muscle portions of beef.

As people got further and further from the soil, had less and less time to cook, or no longer knew what to do with the odds and ends that came from a cow, the demand for things like tongue, thymus, or heart dissolved, and these items disappeared from the grocery store shelf altogether. As we stopped eating glandular and organ meats, we stopped getting the subtle and specialized support nutrients that these parts of the animal offered.

Today many people turn their noses up at gland and organ meats. They would rather take supplements that supply at least some of these important nutritional factors, even though the real thing from the cow does a much better job of supplying usable nutrients. Overall, meats are an excellent source of minerals that are organic. By "organic" I mean that the minerals come from living systems and are part of a matrix of powerful yet subtle nutritional factors, many of which we probably haven't even discovered yet. In addition, the nutrients in meat are ready to use as well as easy to absorb, something we describe as being "bio-available." They are a great way to get high quality amino acids, Vitamins A, D, E, and B-12, along with many trace minerals, zinc, and magnesium.

❖

Over the last few years, there has been a lot of bad press about Creutzfeld-Jacobs disease (CJD), also known as mad cow disease. Some people have blamed the agricultural industry for spreading this disease because of its practice of grinding up already diseased cow parts and processing them into feed proteins for other cows. But evidence kept well hidden from the mainstream points to another very likely origin of the disease.

The most telling evidence is from a man named Mark Purdey who was raising organic beef in England. When cattle in the local area were being attacked and infested with a pest known as the warble fly, the UK government issued a court order that all cattle had to be treated with a pesticide. The pesticide chosen was Phosmet, a powerful organo-phosphate, which was applied along the spine of the cows and allowed to run down their bodies. Mark Purdey refused to comply with the court order to douse his cows with Phosmet as this would have ruined his organic status. He was taken to court but won his case and did not apply the pesticide to his cows.

A short time after the Phosmet baths began, CJD turned up everywhere on farms surrounding the Purdey farm. Although the British government tried to push the theory of a strange new infection somehow rooted in bad feed, Purdey's cows had eaten some of that same feed and showed no signs of coming down with mad cow disease.

Having something of a scientific nature himself, Purdey began to research the problem. He learned that CJD almost always began in the retina of the eye and proceeded from there into the brain. Prions, a form of protein in the retina and spine of mammals, worked as shock absorbers for damaging ultraviolet rays and other oxidizing substances – unless they were damaged by exposure to organophosphates. Once damaged, the prions tended to react with manganese, which turned them into rogue molecules and set off a chain-reaction of tragic destruction in the eye and brain.

Says Fintan Dunne in *Acres, USA* news, "Once this prion defense system is rendered ineffective by organophosphates (the same chemical used to get rid of head lice or scabies in people) there is…an unmediated impact on tissues. Eventually, UV radiation damages the retina, and oxidative stress (goes on from there to) destroy the brain tissues of CJD patients. This theory would expect to find higher CJD incidence in mountain regions, where UV radiation levels are elevated. That prediction holds true." [37]

---

[37] *Acres USA News*, March 2001.

Cambridge University prion bio-chemist David R. Brown is dismissive of the science behind the "infectious" model of CJD, also known as Bovine Spongiform Encephalopathy (BSE), and insists there is "no evidence an infectious agent is present in either meat or milk." And in the U.S., the "Center for Disease Control has conducted experiments on mice that confirm the organophosphate risk."

"The pharmaceutical industry is all the more determined to hide the chemical source of BSE and CJD because a spotlight on chemicals would expose the role the insecticides have in Alzheimer's – another neurodegenerative disease – that might lead to claims which would dwarf those from BSE and CJD litigants." [38]

The message in all of this is that mad cow disease is not some mysterious, vicious infective agent with no known cause. It is the result of a pesticide that damages, then disables, an important defense system in the body, creating mutations that then go on to become very destructive.

Many years ago, not long after Louis Pasteur had discovered bacteria and declared it to be the cause of disease, he, Bernard Claude, a physiologist, and Pierre Bechamp, another chemist, began to argue. Pasteur believed that the bacteria had to be killed or they would invade and create illness. Bernard and Bechamp believed that bacteria were the *result* of disease, not the cause. Bernard declared that the conditions existing in the terrain where the bacteria lived were the all-important determining factors and that the bacteria would not appear if the tissues of the body were healthy.

For the rest of their lives they argued back and forth, Pasteur declaring that the bacteria reigned supreme, whereas Bernard and Bechamp kept insisting that it was the terrain that mattered most.

Although Pasteur won most of the public sympathy during his lifetime, it is said that on his deathbed, he suddenly sat up and said to his family in attendance, "Bernard was right. The microbe is nothing, the *terrain* is everything." [39]

Time has also proven Bernard and Bechamp to be right. The message is, take care of your terrain! ❖

---

[38] *Acres USA News*, March 2001.
[39] Walter McQuade and Ann Aikman, *Stress* (New York, NY: Bantam Books, 1975) p. 18.

10
Milk

WHEN I WAS A LITTLE GIRL, the milkman used to deliver milk to our house two or three times a week. He put the milk, which came in one-quart glass bottles, in a covered metal box on the front porch. The glass bottles had a thick lip around the top edge and a thick layer of cream floating on the milk. I thought having a milkman was extremely modern and sophisticated compared to my grandma, who had to go out and milk her cow, then separate the milk from the cream before putting it in a pitcher in her refrigerator.

Much later, when I was about 12, a large, modern grocery store opened in town. We then began to buy milk in wax-coated cardboard cartons that declared the milk inside to be both "pasteurized" and "homogenized." The milk didn't have any cream floating on the top, and at that time, I thought how convenient it was that we didn't have to take time to shake the bottle every time we wanted to pour a glass of milk.

Today, I have a cow and calf, and every day I milk her then put the fresh, raw milk in a pitcher in the refrigerator.

"Why bother when you can just go to the store and buy it?" people often ask.

Why? Lots of reasons. I want raw milk with all of its enzymes still in it. I want butter made from raw cream. I want fresh, unpasteurized cream on my blueberries and raspberries. I want the prodigious amounts of vitamins and minerals in raw milk. I want the raw, saturated, animal fat in my diet. And I want access to the Wulzen Factor, an anti-stiffness factor discovered by Weston Price that is destroyed during pasteurization. [40] [41]

The process of pasteurization started back in the early 1900s when many people were looking for answers to the unsolved horror of tuberculosis and believed the disease might be coming from cow's milk.

When Louis Pasteur claimed that bacteria were the source of disease and that high temperatures could destroy many forms of bacteria, the authorities suggested that everyone should heat milk to a temperature somewhere between 140 and 180 degrees, a process that came to be known as *pasteurization.*

Although milk is pasteurized to kill harmful bacteria, the process also kills the enzymes that are necessary to help digest and absorb all of the nutrients in the milk. In addition, heating anything to high temperatures denatures proteins. This changes the shape and structure of the protein molecules in milk, rendering them unusable by the body and reducing the nutritional value of it as a food.

As it turned out, milk was not the root cause of TB. The real culprit was a drop in nutrition in both people and animals, which resulted in the immune system's inability to defend the body against the tuberculosis bacteria in many species.

In the days before pasteurization began, a six-month diet of raw, healthy milk was a powerful *healer* of tuberculosis, and those who could afford it went to spend six months or more at "health farms" out in the country where they rested and drank plentiful amounts of milk, cream, cheese, and yogurt. Called "the milk cure," this method of healing disappeared after pasteurization began because pasteurized milk just didn't heal anything.

Today, we know that tuberculosis is just another degenerative disease resulting from poor nutrition. The moment there is a drop in nutrition, there is a decrease in immunity and an increase in susceptibility to bacteria and viruses. This is the degenerative effect that we see everywhere around us. People and animals are all susceptible to TB if the quality of the nutrition they receive falls below a certain level. In cows,

[40] Price, p. 437-458.
[41] Sally Fallon, *Nourishing Traditions* (San Diego, CA: ProMotion Publishing, 1995) p. 15.

tuberculosis is called "brucellosis" or sometimes "Bang's Disease." In our typically aggressive and shortsighted way, we have gone after the disease with chemicals in an effort to suppress the bacteria, instead of correcting the problem of poor nutrition.

Today, cows are tested regularly for bovine tuberculosis, and there is no need to worry about developing the once-mysterious TB. However, by the time the true cause of TB was discovered and a test for it was developed, an entire industry had sprung up to pasteurize milk. The government did not want to put people out of work, and no one really knew the harm that pasteurizing caused, so the processing of milk became a law and continues today, except in California and a handful of other states where a very health- and beauty-conscious population demand that raw milk be made available, and thus it is sold in the stores there.

The tragic loss for the rest of us is that during the heating process the natural enzymes in the milk are destroyed. These are the very enzymes that Mother Nature designed and developed in milk to help our body digest and absorb the nutrients in it.

Without the help of the natural enzymes in raw milk, not only does the pancreas have to work much harder to digest it, it is much more difficult to find anything nutritionally useful in it. Instead of being a healing food, pasteurized milk becomes another irritant, causing allergies, sinus problems, digestive troubles, and mucus in the body. This is why you will so often hear or read the argument that cow's milk is only for calves and is bad for adult humans. The truth is that real (raw) milk is *very* good for you.

❖

Before pasteurization and homogenization began, it was common to sell milk as a whole and unprocessed food. Some cream was removed for making butter or sour cream, but the rest of the milk was consumed whole.

Not long after pasteurizing became common, the milk industry started homogenizing milk. I suspect that those who processed and packaged milk for sale realized that they could separate the cream from the milk and sell a cup of cream for the same price as an entire quart of milk. However, the remaining bit of cream that would rise to the surface of the milk was a clear indication that most of the cream had been removed. Old-timers who knew the power of cream might have objected to this because they used the amount of cream sitting on top of the milk to assess the quality and value of the milk. The more cream, the higher the quality. With homogenization, the fact that there was very little cream sitting on the milk was obscured because homogenization prevented the cream from rising.

Another factor in homogenization may have been the move away from the old breeds of dairy cattle—Jersey, Guernsey, and Brown Swiss—that produced milk with 5-7% cream content, to newer breeds like the Holstein that produce milk with only 2-3% cream. In the old days, this would have been an unacceptable level of cream, and no one would have been able to sell such milk. Homogenization allowed us to disguise the low cream content, and today, 2% and lowfat milk are purchased and consumed without a second thought.

Homogenization is a simple process of shaking or forcing the milk through small tubes so violently that many of the large enzyme molecules present in the milk are shattered into tiny, irregular pieces. People drink the milk and take in the shattered enzymes. These tiny pieces of enzyme then manage to pass into the blood stream where they irritate the walls of veins and arteries. The body's response to this irritation is to produce cholesterol and line the walls of the circulatory system with it in order to protect the tissues from the irritating effects of the broken enzymes.

❖

In the old days, cows were fed and fattened on pasture grass, herbs, and vegetables. Nowadays, cows are fed and fattened on corn and soy crops containing the residues of toxic chemicals and heavy metals. These toxins have a great affinity for fat cells, and the fat in cows' milk can pick up these toxins, passing them on to the humans who drink the milk.

When milk causes digestive upsets, allergies, gas, and sinus problems, it *may* be because an individual does not produce the specific enzymes necessary to digest milk and milk fats. But more often, it is because pasteurization has destroyed its protein structures, homogenization has shattered a key enzyme that then becomes an irritant, and the whole mess carries a load of toxins and chemicals because pesticides and heavy metals are drawn to the fat in milk.

When a farmer milks cows, the milk is picked up from the bulk tank and delivered to a milk-processing factory. Once there, it is broken down into its basic constituents – water, milk solids, light cream and heavy cream. Next it is pasteurized, then homogenized and put back together using carefully controlled recipes depending on whether the goal is skim milk, 2% milk, or whole milk. When the milk has been reassembled, a few synthetic vitamins and minerals may be added, and sometimes a little instant milk powder to give the milk a little more body and color. Once milk has gone through this process, it's hard to consider it as milk at all anymore.

The loss of the nutritional powerhouse that milk used to be has contributed to the subtle processes of degeneration in millions of people. With increasingly poor nutrition, bile production in the liver and gall bladder is reduced. Without plenty of bile to emulsify fats, we are unable to utilize these fats, and without fats you will be unable to absorb and use vitamins A, D, E, and K – the fat-soluble vitamins that are the necessary basics for any kind of healing.

For a long time, I drank almost no milk. Today, I know the healing power of milk in its whole, raw, unprocessed forms. Raw, unpasteurized milk, cream, butter, sour cream, and cheeses do not cause allergies, asthma, ear-nose-and-throat problems, high cholesterol, heart disease, or many of the other difficulties blamed on dairy products. These problems are the result of degenerative processes in the body caused by poor nutrition in the first place. Pasteurized milk will aggravate these conditions by clogging up the body, the sinuses, lungs, ears, nose, and throat with mucus, which becomes a perfect breeding ground for bacteria. The lactic-acid-producing bacteria that keep you safe from certain pathogens is destroyed when milk is pasteurized. Over half its water-soluble vitamins are lost, proteins become less available, and minerals, which are many, are changed in subtle ways that make them inorganic and more difficult to assimilate.

Real, raw milk does not create these problems. Whole, unpasteurized, unhomogenized milk comes complete with high levels of nutrition plus all the enzymes and digestive factors that are necessary for you to digest that milk.

My granddaughter cannot drink commercially processed, "store-bought" milk at all. When she does, her eyes swell and dark circles – the telltale allergy bull's-eyes – appear under them. After a week on the pasteurized stuff, her sinuses are swollen, her nose is plugged up; she sneezes, wheezes, and suffers. However, these problems disappear when she drinks the whole, raw milk our cows produce here at the farm. Not only do problems disappear, but her good health and high energy reappear.

Remember, good health is not just an *absence* of symptoms; it is the *presence* of high energy, endless stamina, creative intelligence, an interest in work, and a peaceful disposition.

A cup of raw milk on my oatmeal in the morning, a couple of tablespoons of butter on my muffin at noon, a dish of homemade yogurt, and a chunk of cheese as an afternoon or evening snack have brought a smoothness to my skin, a shine and fullness to my hair, firm strength to my fingernails, stable weight loss, the disappearance of cravings, and a tremendous sense of well-being. ❖

11
Fats and Cholesterol

NOTHING IS MORE misunderstood in the modern diet than fat. Every month, the popular press turns out warnings about the dangers of eating fat. Everywhere you look you are urged to eat non-fat or low-fat foods, to use polyunsaturated vegetable oils, and if possible, to eliminate fats. Animal fats and saturated fats are expressly named as the culprit in all manner of diseases from heart attacks and high cholesterol to cancers, obesity, and atherosclerosis.

I have had some people nearly faint away when they hear the truth about fat. They think they have been doing everything right to maintain their good health...eating no meat, drinking no milk, avoiding fat, eating lots of whole grains and soy products. When they end up with a catastrophic illness and have done everything they can to no avail, they often find their way to my classes and are shocked to discover that what they thought was the correct way to eat has greatly contributed to, or even caused, their illness.

The facts of the matter are that you not only need fat in your diet, you need saturated animal fats, as well as *super*unsaturated fats, and you should avoid polyunsaturated fats in almost all forms. When you think of fats, think in terms of what you need to take in for your body's sake, not in terms of what you need to avoid. One of the worst things you can do is eliminate fats from your diet.

Fat molecules are made of carbon atoms strung together in a chain, with one or more hydrogen atoms along the length of the chain. Fats come in a variety of forms and each form has different uses in the body. Short-chain and medium-chain fats create quick energy. They also have anti-microbial, anti-fungal, and anti-tumor properties, as well as an ability to enhance growth and improve the function of the immune system.

Long-chain fats and extra-long-chain fats are needed for building tissues and cell membranes as well as producing hemoglobin, cholesterol, and other hormone-like substances. Long-chain fats are also necessary for absorption into the lymph system, for velvety skin, vitality, and fast healing power. They can lower blood pressure if it is high and raise it if it is low, create a sense of stamina and calm, and help generate needed electrical currents that drive chemical transactions in the body.

Butter contains mostly short- and medium-chain fats, as does coconut oil, both of which are good for you. Olive oil, a *mono*-unsaturated fat that is somewhat usable in the body, is mostly long-chain fats, as are fish oils and flaxseed oil.

Beef and pork both contain saturated fats having a range of short- to long-chain fats, but are mostly long-chain.

Your brain is 55% fat, and you need fats in your diet to help your brain run smoothly and well. Mother's breast milk is over 50% saturated fat and is critical for development of the brain and central nervous system in the newborn and young child. [42]

Researchers have found that putting children on low-fat or soy milk diets not only interferes with brain development, it results in allergies, learning disorders, attention deficit disorders, hyperkinetic behaviors, and other mental, emotional, and social problems in children. One of several problems with soy is that it does not have the fat so desperately required by the developing human brain. Another is that it deranges the endocrine system. [43] [44]

Several years ago, pediatricians of America issued a statement saying they believed that soymilk formulas were not appropriate for infants, and that such formulas had contributed to the epidemic of ADHD

---

[42] Udo Erasmus, *Fats that Heal, Fats that Kill* (Burnaby, BC, Canada: Alive Books, 1993) p. 50-51.
[43] Gary Null PhD, *Nutrition and The Mind* (New York, NY: Four Walls Eight Windows Press, 1995) p. 225.
[44] Fallon, *The Oiling of America,* 1998.

children. I heard this on a National Public Radio (NPR) news program and was thrilled that the truth was now out in public. But that was the last that was heard on the subject. We are still not paying attention to what we are doing with food.

❖

Adults have come to believe that eating saturated animal fats will cause high cholesterol, high triglycerides, atherosclerosis, and similar diseases. But these problems are not caused by eating fat; *they are the result of poor nutrition coupled with eating sugar, skeletonized foods, and stress.*

The belief that fats cause heart disease, cancer, and other diseases is known as *The Lipid Hypothesis*. This theory started back in the 1950s when a researcher named Ancel Keys not only did some very poor research, he also came to an erroneous conclusion. Once published, however, others jumped on the bandwagon and began to undertake biased, lopsided, already-prejudiced research. Some of this research was funded by the budding vegetable oil producers who needed a reason backed by "scientific research" to convince people it was a good idea to switch from traditional fats – the butter, lard, and tallow that we had used safely for thousands of years – to the new, factory-made, imitation fats known as margarine and corn oil. Once this faulty research was published, the food factories began serious marketing campaigns and succeeded in getting millions to change their diets to the "new and improved" foods they were producing. [45] [46]

Fortunately, we are beginning to wake up in terms of our need for healthy fats. Even the famous Framingham Study in Massachusetts, which tracked thousands of people for 40 years, reversed its position recently, saying, "The more saturated fat one ate, the more cholesterol one ate, the more calories one ate, the lower the person's serum cholesterol (was). We found that the people who ate the most cholesterol, ate the most saturated fat, ate the most calories, weighed the least and were the most physically active." [47]

Numerous other studies indicate that when saturated fats and cholesterol are reduced, there is only a *very* marginal reduction in heart

[45] Uffe Ravnskov MD, PhD, *The Cholesterol Myths* (Washington, DC: New Trends Publishing Inc, 2000) p. 15-16
[46] Fallon, *The Oiling of America,* 1998.
[47] Fallon, *The Oiling of America,* 1998.

disease, whereas deaths from all other causes go *up*, including cancer, stroke, suicide, brain hemorrhage, and even violent deaths.[48] [49]

Another thing that simply must be understood about fats is that when you eat sweets and processed grains or foods made with either of these, for example white and whole wheat flour, rice, pasta, many common breakfast cereals, or any kind of sugar, whether in candies, cookies, cakes, syrups, soft drinks, shakes, or some other food, *these foods will be turned into saturated fats by your body.*[50]

The important, enzyme-rich, saturated fats needed by the body and found in such foods as whole raw milk, raw cream, raw butter, and meats have all been cast into the category of forbidden foods that are likely to kill you, while the real culprits – processed foods and refined sugar – are ignored and continue to be advertised as something that will make you feel good, sexy, or part of the "in crowd." Our entire population has been seduced into eating boxed, canned, fast foods, and food-look-alikes composed of tasteless chemicals and white flour, which have been made palatable by the addition of sugar. The result is rampant atherosclerosis, heart disease, high blood pressure, diabetes, and a long list of other diseases.

Udo Erasmus, who studied fats intensely after being dangerously exposed to carcinogenic chemicals, knew their affinity for fats and states bluntly, "Killer saturated long-chain fatty acids, which are sticky and therefore increase our chances of stroke, heart attack, clogged arteries, and diabetes, are produced from refined sugars." [51]

Cholesterol, another supposed "bad boy," is actually a very important healing agent in the body. Cholesterol is manufactured in the liver, and the body uses it to protect tissues and manage the fluidity/hardness of cell membranes, thus controlling what gets into or out of your cells. Most male and female sex hormones are made from cholesterol, as are other hormones that regulate conditions such as water balance in the kidneys, the stress response, the strength of artery walls, and many other functions. Vitamin D is made from cholesterol. So are bile acids. Cholesterol is part of a light covering on the skin that keeps it from drying out, and it even works as an anti-oxidant when the body is short of these.

---

[48] Fallon, *The Oiling of America,* 1998.
[49] Ravnskov, p. 30-31.
[50] Erasmus, p. 31-32.
[51] Erasmus, pg. 34.

Problems with cholesterol arise when you do not have enough of the right materials available for the body's continuous rebuilding needs – especially the right kinds of saturated and unsaturated essential fats (essential fatty acids are often called EFAs) that work hand-in-hand with proteins.

When the body does not have enough building materials to build good structure, it will begin to skimp when rebuilding body structures such as bones, teeth, organs, and artery walls. If these structures get too thin, the body will then produce extra cholesterol to temporarily "plaster" the insides of thin or weak artery walls, veins, or organs, shoring them up in an effort to strengthen them. In the case of arteries, this helps prevent them from leaking, breaking, or bulging out to form aneurysms, but it also prevents the normal and natural expansion and contraction of the arteries and veins. The result is a rigid cardiovascular system, creating a condition that we call "high blood pressure" or "hypertension."

Besides low nutrition and high sugar, the most dangerous factor in raising your cholesterol is a constant level of physical or emotional stress. Too much cholesterol will also be produced whenever you take in more calories than you can burn off, regardless of the source of those calories. The bottom line is that you need to manage and balance the fats in your diet. Too little fat is worse than too much. Too little cholesterol is worse than too much because true research – not the fake, manipulated kind – shows that, as cholesterol goes down, the incidence of heart attack is lowered minimally while the incidence of cancer goes up. [52]

In her book, *Nourishing Traditions,* author Sally Fallon discusses cholesterol saying, "When thyroid function is poor, often the result of a diet high in sugar and low in nutrients, the body floods the blood with cholesterol as an adaptive and protective mechanism, providing a superabundance of the materials needed to heal tissues and produce protective steroids. Just as a large police force is needed in a locality where crime occurs frequently, cholesterol is needed in a poorly nourished body to protect the individual from a tendency to heart disease and cancer. Blaming coronary heart disease on cholesterol is like blaming the police for murder and theft in a high crime area." [53]

Fallon also illuminates Dr. Nathan Pritikin's famous fat-free Pritikin Diet and the results for those who followed it. "Those who possessed enough will power to stay fat-free for any length of time

---

[52] Ravnskov, p.145, 208, 210, 218.
[53] Fallon, *Nourishing Traditions,* p. 11.

developed a variety of health problems including low energy, difficulty in concentrating, depression, weight gain, and signs of mineral deficiencies. Pritikin may have saved himself from heart disease, but his low-fat diet did not spare him from cancer. He died, in the prime of life, of leukemia." [54]

Fallon points out that if you step back to look at the bigger picture surrounding the issue of fat intake, you will see that as consumption of animal fats went down, and the consumption of polyunsaturated vegetable oils went up, so did heart disease, cancers, depression, suicides, and violence in society. When you put several statistical curves next to each other, one for the increasing use of vegetable oils, one for increasing heart disease, and one for increasing cancer, the curves run almost parallel to one another. [55] [56]

Saturated fat is so important in the diet that it is difficult to see and hear it get beaten up in the popular press again and again. Many people, even scientists, confuse saturated animal fats with *hydrogenated* fats. A natural, saturated animal fat like beef tallow or lard is solid at room temperature and fairly stable, even at high cooking temperatures. Lots of people think that shortening is saturated animal fat. It is not. Shortening is vegetable oil that has been turned into a solid, hydrogenated fat. The process of hydrogenation is so destructive that I quote a small section from Sally Fallon's *Nourishing Traditions*:

"**Hydrogenation:** This is the process that turns polyunsaturates, normally liquid at room temperature, into a fat that is solid at room temperature – margarine and shortening. To produce them, manufacturers begin with the cheapest oils – soy, corn or cottonseed – already rancid from the extraction process. These oils are then mixed with tiny metal particles – usually nickel oxide. Nickel oxide is very toxic when absorbed and is impossible to totally eliminate from the margarine. The oil with its nickel catalyst is then subjected to hydrogen gas in a high pressure, high temperature reactor. Next, soap-like emulsifiers and starch are squeezed into the mixture to give it a better consistency; the oil is yet

[54] Fallon, *Nourishing Traditions*, p. 4.
[55] Fallon, *The Oiling of America*, 1998.
[56] Erasmus, p. 111.

again subjected to high temperature when it is steam-cleaned. This removes its horrible odor. Margarine's natural color, an unappetizing grey, is removed by bleach. Coal-tar dyes and strong (artificial) flavors must then be added to make it resemble butter. Finally the mixture is compressed and packaged in blocks or tubs, ready to be spread on your toast.

"Margarine and other partially hydrogenated oils are even worse for you than the highly refined vegetable oils from which they are made, because of chemical changes that occur during the hydrogenation process. Under high temperatures, the nickel catalyst causes the hydrogen atoms to change position on the fatty acid chain. Before hydrogenation, two hydrogen atoms occur together on the chain, causing the chain to bend slightly and creating an electron cloud at the site of the double bond. This is called the *cis* formation, the configuration most commonly found in nature. With hydrogenation, one hydrogen atom is moved to the other side so that the molecule straightens. This is called the *trans* con-figuration, rarely found in nature. These man-made *trans*fats are toxins to the body. But unfortunately your digestive system does not recognize them as such. Instead of being eliminated, the *trans*fats are incorporated into the body's cell membranes as if they were *cis*fats – and your cells actually become hydrogenated! Once in place, *trans*fatty acids with their misplaced hydrogen atom wreak havoc in cell metabolism. These altered fats actually block the utilization of essential fatty acids, causing many deleterious effects ranging from sexual dysfunction to increased blood cholesterol and paralysis of the immune system.

"In the 1940s, researchers found a strong correlation between cancer and the consumption of fat – the fats used were hydrogenated fats, not naturally saturated (animal) fats. (Until recently, the confusion between hydrogenated fats and naturally saturated fats has persisted not only in the popular press, but in scientific databases, resulting in much error in study results.)

Consumption of hydrogenated fats is associated with a host of other serious diseases, not only cancer but also atherosclerosis, diabetes, obesity, immune system dysfunction, low birth weight babies and birth defects, sterility, difficulty in lactation and problems with bones and tendons; yet hydrogenated fats continue to be promoted as health foods. Margarine's popularity represents a triumph of advertising duplicity over common sense. Your best defense is to avoid it like the plague." [57]

Let's have a very short course in fats, putting the facts out there as simply and clearly as possible.

Your body is made of cells. Each cell is enclosed by what is called a cell membrane. The cell membrane is composed of a double layer of fats. This double layer is constructed by weaving together a variety of fatty acid chains, some of them saturated, some unsaturated. The saturated fats tend to be straight and stick-like in form. They pack together very tightly and can create an impenetrable wall. The *mono*unsaturated fats have a slight kink in them, which prevents such tight packing. The *poly*unsaturated fats have two kinks in them making them almost L-shaped. The *super*unsaturated fats have 3 kinks in them which makes them almost C-shaped and it is this C-shape which proves to be so important in the construction of cell membranes simply because the C-shaped molecules do not pack together very well. This allows the cell membrane to retain more fluidity, respond better to its environment, open to admit nutrients or eliminate toxins, and close to prevent invasion by bacteria, viruses, pesticides, or other unwanted substances.

In addition to the looser packing allowed by *super*unsaturated fats, the kinks in their molecular chains are created by two hydrogen atoms sitting next to each other. These adjacent charges create differences in electrical potential and these, in turn, create electrical currents, which help to drive chemical transactions in and around the cell. The more transactions your cells can manage, the healthier you will be.

The bottom line is…

- There are saturated fats, and there are unsaturated fats.

- You *need* both saturated and unsaturated fats in your diet.

[57] Fallon, *Nourishing Traditions,* p. 12-13.

- No less than 20% of your calories should come from fats.

- The needed balance between fats in your body is about one-third saturated fats, one-third monounsaturated fats, and one-third superunsaturated fats.

- In the saturated fats category, there are:

  o Short-chain fats found in butter, known as butyric acid.

  o Medium-chain fats found in coconut, palm, and palm kernel oils, all known as palmitic acid.

  o Longer-chain fats found in beef, lamb, mutton, pork, butter, and cocoa butter.

- Saturated fats are very stable even at high cooking temperatures, thus the danger of *trans*-fats is avoided.

- The body burns short- and medium-chain saturated fats as a major source of quick, long-lasting energy.

- The body uses medium- and long-chain saturated fats to build structures, make some energy, construct cell membranes, and make small amounts of *poly*unsaturated fatty acids for its own use.

- Of the unsaturated fats, there are 3 kinds: *mono*unsaturated, *poly*unsaturated, and *super*unsaturated.

- *Mono*unsaturated fats with a slight kink and one double bond are found in olives, almonds, avocadoes, peanuts, pecans, cashews, filberts, and macadamia nuts, and the oils of all these.

- *Poly*unsaturated fats have two double bonds, thus, two kinks, and are found in safflower, sunflower, hemp, walnut, pumpkin, sesame, and flaxseed oils.

- *Super*unsaturated fats have three or more double bonds, thus, three kinks, and are found in flax seeds, hemp seeds, walnut oil, and dark green leaves.

- The most important unsaturated fats for humans are the superunsaturated fats.

- The superunsaturated fats are rich in Omega 3 and Omega 6 oils.

- In the body, the Omega 3 and Omega 6 oils are known as *essential fatty acids*, (EFAs) which means the body cannot make them, they must be supplied.

- Omega 3 oil is sometimes known as Alpha-Linolenic Acid, and flaxseed oil is the richest source.

- Omega 6 oil is sometimes known as Linoleic Acid, and the richest sources are safflower, sunflower, and hempseed oil.

- Another important form of Omega 6 oil is called Gamma-Linolenic Acid and is found mainly in borage, black currant, and evening primrose oils.

- A third form of Omega 6 oil, called Arachidonic Acid (AA), is found in meats and animal products such as milk, cheese, etc.

- Omega 3 and Omega 6 oils must be supplied to the body in a 1:3 ratio. This means approximately 1,000 mg of Omega 3 for every 3,000 mg of Omega 6. For health maintenance, if you need 2,000 – 3,000 mg of Omega 3 oil per day, then you would need 6,000 – 9,000 mg of Omega 6 oil per day. This would be a balanced ratio of superunsaturated oils in your diet.

- Hempseed oil is the best source of unsaturated EFAs because it contains the correct ratio of Omega 3 to Omega 6 oil.

- All of the unsaturated fats are very unstable and tend to react quickly, making it necessary to have a good supply of antioxidants in the body at all times.

- Light is the biggest enemy of unsaturated fats. Any oils you buy should come in cans or dark, light-proof bottles.

- Almost as a matter of course, the fatty acid chains in *poly*unsaturated vegetable oils are seriously damaged during processing, making them useless and harmful to us. They quickly become rancid when exposed to light, oxygen, or heat. Rancid oils *seek and destroy* vitamins A and D in the body.

- If you do not have fats in your diet, you will not be able to use vitamins A, D, E, and K because these are oil-soluble vitamins. If you cannot use vitamin A, you simply will not heal. And conversely, without vitamin A, the essential fatty acids will not work. Without Vitamin D you will not be able to utilize calcium, which means your bones will degenerate. Without E you will have difficulties with skin, cardiovascular function, and healing. And without Vitamin K you will not be able to maintain healthy bones, heart function, and resistance to aging.

❖

The point of all of the above is that you absolutely must have good quality fats in your diet, both saturated and unsaturated. What's more, they must be available in the right proportions.

The saturated fats you eat are best for you when they are eaten raw, and the best source of raw saturated animal fat is raw butter, milk, or cream. The richest source of unsaturated Omega 3 fat is flaxseed oil, which also contains some Omega 6. The richest source of unsaturated Omega 6 fat is safflower oil, however, most safflower oil is rancid from processing and exposure to light in the clear bottles it is packaged in. The best source of both Omega 3 and 6 in one oil is hempseed oil, because it carries them in the correct proportions of one part Omega 3 to three parts Omega 6 oil. You can also get some Omega 3 and 6 oils by including *raw* nuts such as walnuts, pecans, cashews, almonds, and plenty of dark green leaves such as kale, collards, dark lettuces, and lambsquarter in your salads.

Hempseed oil can be found at your local health food store. If you have difficulty finding it, use flaxseed oil. A good way to get both the Omega 3 and 6 essential fats into your diet is to put 1-2 TBSP of flaxseed oil on your tossed salad every day, then pour your regular oil-and-vinegar, Italian, or Ranch dressing right over top of the flaxseed oil to cover the taste, which is somewhat bitter. Be sure to eat/sip all the dressing in the bottom of the salad plate. If you can get hempseed oil, use the same amount, 1-2 TBSP on your salad and cover the taste with your regular dressing.

For these essential unsaturated fats to work in your body, you must also be sure to take vitamins A, C, B3, B6, E, beta carotene, and the minerals magnesium and zinc.

Do not avoid saturated animal fats as if they are the plague.

Do not use commercial vegetable oils that were produced with high temperatures or in lighted pressing facilities. This is even more important if they are Omega 3 and 6 oils. And anything in clear glass or plastic bottles that exposes the oil to light will be rancid and very harmful to you. Oils react first to light, then to oxygen, and lastly to heat.

Do not cook with vegetable oils, they are too unstable. As a general rule try not to fry your foods because extremely high temperatures will denature fats and proteins. If you have a hankering for something fried, use bacon fat, lard, or beef tallow because these are very stable. When you fry, use the lowest frying temperature possible.

Do eat butter. If you have access to butter made from raw, unpasteurized cream, enjoy it even more freely. If it is raw butter, try to eat at least two tablespoons per day as a minimum, although four to eight tablespoons would be more acceptable.

Do enjoy ice cream if you make it yourself using raw milk or cream.

Do eat beef, pork, chicken, mutton, fish, and other meats because they are good for you, but don't overdose, especially if you're still eating sugar or if you don't know who raised the animals and how they were fed.

Do use olive oil or peanut oil (both *mono*unsaturated) in small amounts to make salad dressings if they have been cold pressed in a dark workroom and you buy it in a can or dark bottle that the light cannot get through. Otherwise, the body does not have much use for *mono*unsaturated fats, and even less use for *poly*unsaturated fats because it will make its own versions when needed. ❖

12
Grains & Legumes
(aka Pulses)

IF YOU ARE LIKE MANY people, you don't think about grain as grain, you think of it as bread or cereal, pasta or pumpernickel, chips or granola, baked beans, pea soup, or something else. Although grains and legumes have many vitamins and minerals in them in their natural, unprocessed state, once the food processing industry has turned them into the breads, cereals, and other foods that you are familiar with, they have been almost completely stripped of their nutrients.

When you eat anything made with white flour, not only do you *not* get the vitamins, minerals, wheat germ oils, and enzymes that Mother Nature put in the wheat, your body has to supply many chemical and nutritional elements from its reserve stock in order to digest and metabolize these over-refined grain skeletons. In other words, your body has to spend a little of its energy in the hopes of being able to replace this energy and get the bonus of whatever was in the food. When there is nothing in the food, the body comes up short. It's like putting money in a savings account and then discovering that, not only did you not collect any interest, the bank charged you a recurring fee for holding your money.

Nowadays, the most common grains include wheat, oats, rye, and rice. A few less common are barley, spelt, millet, amaranth, and kamut. There are others, but unless you're really a health food store devotee or highly allergic to the common grains, you may not know that other grains are out there or what you might do with them.

Birds are the only creatures that can actually eat, digest, and benefit from grains in their whole, natural, dry state. Some mammals have three or four stomachs to allow for proper fermentation processes in digesting grains. However, if humans wish to benefit nutritionally from whole, unrefined grains, the grains must be soaked or sprouted, and breads must be made with old-fashioned sourdough. Otherwise, substances known as phytates, or phytic acids, in the whole grain will bind with calcium, iron, phosphorus, zinc and the other minerals in it, making these important minerals unavailable to you and contributing to physical degeneration.

Someone once asked me if this meant she had to soak her cornflakes and eat soggy cereal every morning, which caused a laugh in class. Cornflakes and other cereals on the grocery store shelf are not whole, they are highly processed. Soaking grains that have already been processed and made into something like corn flakes or a boxed cereal is not necessary...but then eating these highly refined grains does not get you the nutrition you need either. This includes many forms of crackers, corn chips, and other grain-based snack foods. Add rancid, polyunsaturated, and hydrogenated oils, along with a little refined white sugar, and you have a real witch's brew.

One way to enjoy grains with *all* of their vitamins, minerals, oils, and enzymes is to make and eat 14-Grain Cereal. To make a batch of it, you will need 1 lb. (approximately 1 cup) of each of the following grains. Keep in mind that whole grains are often referred to as "berries."

14-Grain Cereal

Whole wheat berries	Flax seeds
Whole oat berries	Popcorn
Whole rye berries	Buckwheat
Barley	Millet
Mung bean seeds	Lentils
Alfalfa seeds	Brown rice
Sesame seeds	Almonds

Put these grains into a large bowl or pot that will allow you to mix the dry grains without spilling them all over. Mix well and store in quart jars with lids. You will need about four quart jars for one batch of

14-Grain Cereal. Put three of the jars in your freezer for later use, and put the last one in your refrigerator.

After supper each night, put 2-4 TBSP of the mixed grains into a small grinder. Small grain grinders can be purchased for about $20 at a discount store. Popular brands include Salton and West Bend, and there are probably others.

Grind for about 30 seconds, then stop and look at the grains. If the popcorn is still fairly large, grind for another 30 seconds. Repeat once or twice more until the popcorn grains are smaller and less discernable. Don't grind too long and hard or the heat generated by the grinding will destroy the enzymes in the grain.

Then pour the ground grain mix into a cereal bowl. Pour about 1 cup of organic apple (or peach, or grape) juice over the ground-up grains and stir. Set a saucer or piece of plastic wrap over the bowl and put in the refrigerator overnight or for *at least eight hours.*

In the morning, just stir and eat. You can add a bit of fresh or frozen fruit to it if you like. In the winter, you can warm it up a little in a larger bowl of hot water, but don't heat too much (don't go over 117°) or you'll destroy enzymes. There are lots of variations on this cereal. Some people just soak the grains in water, some soak them in milk with a couple tablespoons of yogurt added, some use water, yogurt, and salt. In the morning, they add maple syrup or raw honey and fruit. If you can't handle the fruit juice because of diabetes, try the yogurt combination. Eating 14-Grain Cereal three or four times a week will provide you with a tremendous boost in nutrition. If you had to survive on this cereal for a long period of time, it would supply all the vitamins, minerals, and amino acids your body needs.

Everything your body does is based on being able to get a steady supply of glucose. Your body needs these *natural* sugars in *whole* forms that break down slowly and don't suddenly overdose your system with sugar, which upsets the balance between your liver, pancreas, and adrenals. Whole grains and legumes are good sources of carbohydrates that break down slowly into sugars and starches for the body's use.

Refined white sugar, brown sugar (which is really white sugar sprayed with a little molasses), corn syrup, sucrose, fructose, and dextrose are some of the common names for what is really a very dangerous substance as far as your body is concerned. Sugar deranges your endocrine system and unbalances body chemistry. It was originally used as a tranquilizer and sedative.

Only one hundred years ago, smoking opium was acceptable, whereas eating refined sugar was considered to be a despicable addiction. [58] People went to jail or were run out of town for adding sugar to beer or bread, thus, ruining what were considered to be two important staples of life. [59] Today's beer and bread are nothing like their counterparts of a few centuries ago. Back then, these foods contributed to good health; today, they ruin good health.

A few centuries ago, a pound of sugar cost a year's worth of wages and only the very rich could afford it. Sugar is so highly addictive that those who first tasted it immediately craved more of it, and soon the rich, along with their servants who had sneaked a bit from the pantry, began to suffer from the strange disease called diabetes, along with physical, mental, and emotional difficulties that had never been seen before.

Today, you will sometimes hear doctors and other medical people say that there is no known cause of diabetes and that even Hippocrates was puzzled by the disease. They then go on to point out that this was back in the days before the use of sugar. However, this is not only untrue, it is shortsighted and misleading. Sugar addiction and its diseases were rampant among the Arabic and Islamic peoples of the Middle East. [60] Hippocrates was famed for his healing abilities and likely saw the wealthy people from around the Mediterranean who could afford both the high cost of sugar and the trip to his healing clinic. *If* he was not able to discern the cause of diabetes, it may have been because he was not as familiar with sugar in his own culture.

Sugar, one of the sweet spoils of war, was brought steadily westward by a series of invading armies and their conquests. It is widely believed that Christian soldiers were able to stop the Islamic invaders simply because the Turks, Moors, and Saracens had become tired and lost their ferociousness through use of sugared drinks and candied foods. In fact, the 14th century Crusades were planned and carried out with a mission of capturing the sugar technology of the Moslems in order to get a piece of the market in sugar trade and the taxes on it. Christendom did not enjoy obvious military successes with their Crusades, but they succeeded in getting their hands on sugar processing and its lucrative

---

[58] William Dufty, *Sugar Blues* (New York, NY: Warner Books Inc, 1975) p. 41
[59] Dufty, p. 51.
[60] Dufty, p. 30.

potential, and that was enough to satisfy them. Thus, sugar was introduced into European society over the 14th and 15th centuries. [61]

Today, sugar is a major culprit behind many of our worst difficulties because of our ignorance about real food and because people keep choosing sugar-laden, factory-made foods over the simple, natural foods grown by Mother Nature. Without top quality nutrition to maintain high immunity, we end up with heart disease, diabetes, anorexia, depression, dental cavities, multiple sclerosis, poor eyesight, allergies, headache, chronic fatigue, inability to concentrate, alcoholism, obesity, tuberculosis, high cholesterol and triglycerides, digestive problems, atherosclerosis and arteriosclerosis, arthritis, a tendency toward violent behavior, osteoporosis, and especially cancers. Tumors of all kinds love sugar.

Powerful sugar cartels are happy to leave the blame for heart disease, high blood pressure, cancers, and their accompanying disorders at the door of fats. In an effort to market their wares more broadly, the vegetable oil processors inadvertently aided the sugar cartels by advertising their oils as the answer to "the saturated fat problem" when, in truth, rancid vegetable oils and sugar make a lethal combination. By refusing to look honestly at our diet and what has happened to food, we blame many diseases and disorders on genes – and the sugar-based diet is completely ignored.

For all of these reasons, the pharmaceutical and supplement producers are doing some brisk business these days, and no one is looking at the fact that every single food we eat is processed to death before it reaches the grocery store shelves. During the processing, everything we need to survive and thrive in a long, healthy, productive life is removed from the food. Some food processors try to fortify the dead food with a few vitamins and minerals that are just as useless as the food they are added to because they were synthesized in a laboratory and are incompatible with the body's systems.

It is difficult for people to get off of sugar when so many of today's foods are simply an unpalatable mix of chemicals whose taste is covered by sugar. You would not even consider eating this stuff if the sugar didn't cover up the taste of the chemicals, making it so addictive and attractive to your tongue.

When you think about the fact that very little of what we call food today actually has the nutritional supplies that the body requires to

---

[61] Dufty, p. 31.

keep repairing and rebuilding itself, it's a wonder we are all still walking, breathing, and working.

Compounding the "non-food" food problem is the fact that very few people really know how to cook from scratch anymore. Those who do know how have difficulty finding the time for it. We have been duped into working for money in order to buy the necessities of life instead of just making or growing our own. Caught up in glitzy marketing campaigns that create an ever-expanding set of needs, we work, work, work, then shop, shop, shop in a rat's maze of consumerism.

Someday our civilization may be known as the people who became extinct because they insisted on turning everything into a business and money-making venture. Then, when they couldn't afford their own system, they collapsed and died because no one knew how to grow their own food or fiber any more! ❖

13
Organic Vegetables & Fruits

WHEN YOU GO INTO any ordinary grocery store or market today, you will see a large assortment of vegetables and fruits in the produce section. Quite often, they are big, shiny with wax, and tough as shoe leather. When you bite into them, they do not have the rich, velvety taste and sweet juice of healthy, mature fruits.

The plastic bags that hold lettuces and other vegetables can have mild fungicides on the inside of the plastic to keep the vegetables from becoming moldy. Even so, all too often, fresh fruits and vegetables rot and turn to slime within days of purchase.

If you were to go into an organic market, the fresh fruit and vegetable section is not nearly as extensive or impressive. The fruits frequently look small, dry, shrunken, and completely unappetizing. They, too, have very little juice inside, and when you buy them and take them home, they don't last any longer than commercially grown fruits and vegetables. They don't taste any better either, and sometimes they taste worse.

The biggest reason for many dry, shrunken foods in the organic world is the failure of organic producers to restore their soil to a living condition. A good many organic growers simply switch from using chemical pesticides, herbicides, and fungicides to using their "approved" and more natural organic counterparts. In other words, the strategy is the same…plant seeds, then just try to keep the plants growing and upright long enough to produce a fruit and get it to market. Nutritional quality is seldom thought of.

Remember what was said about cows getting too much potassium instead of calcium? The same thing happens in plants. When calcium in the soil is minimal or present, but chemically unavailable because of pH conditions and other bonding issues, the plant will uptake potassium as a replacement for calcium. In a plant, too much potassium causes the plant to produce lots of big, lush leaves, making it look healthy and green. This appearance is deceptive because without the right minerals, the plants and fruits are weak, sick, and bloated.

Overloaded with water, yet without enough calcium and the other minerals needed to build good structure and maintain the energies required for the hundreds of chemical reactions that produce healthy fruit, these are the plants that need serious "propping up" with pesticides, fungicides, and herbicides. Often, growers pick the swollen, tasteless fruit early, before the plant succumbs to mold, mildew, or other disease.

Perhaps you have seen the swollen legs of sick people suffering from heart and circulatory diseases. It's the same thing with plants, except that plants do not have heart attacks, and they will continue to struggle with all their might to produce a fruit that will contain at least a few viable seeds so that their existence will go on through their offspring.

When you are buying fruits and vegetables, ask yourself what kind of soil those fruits might have been raised in. Be aware of the following quality scale that goes from lowest nutrition and quality to highest nutrition and quality:

1. **Commercial** – Foods raised in commercial fields or greenhouses with dead soils and using NPK fertilizers. These will often be big, bright, waxy, tasteless, and have the texture of cardboard. Sometimes they will be mealy; almost always they lack the inner juices full of natural sugars. They will carry a load of pesticides, fungicides, and heavy metals, and be low in vitamins and minerals. They will not taste good when you buy them and will not last long after you get them home, even when kept in a refrigerated environment.

2. **Transitional Organic** – Foods raised in fields or greenhouses in which the farmer has stopped spraying pesticides and fungicides, but has not restored the soil. There may be traces of poisonous chemicals used in previous years. The fungicide Captan can be detected at levels high enough to cause rejection in organic markets 17 years after a farmer

stops using it. Again, the food will be very low in vitamins, minerals, and brix. They also need refrigeration and do not last or store well.

3. **Certified Organic/No Soil Restoration** – Foods raised in fields or greenhouses in which no poisonous chemicals or NPK fertilizers have been used for at least 3-5 years, but the soil has not been restored, and therefore the nutrition in the vegetable or fruit is low. Organic veggies and fruits grown in poor soil without the use of NPK fertilizers often look small and shrunken, and the food will often be just as dry, tasteless, and lacking in vitamins and minerals as commercial foods yet cost much more.

4. **Certified Organic/Some Soil Restoration** – These are foods raised in fields or greenhouses in which there has been an effort to restore the soil to living status. Poisonous chemicals are not used, the use of compost as fertilizer is common along with paramagnetic rock for re-mineralization. Alternative means of managing pests and weeds produces foods that have some vitamins, minerals, and amino acids in them, as well as better taste and much better shelf life.

5. **Bio-Dynamic**® – Organic foods certified by the Demeter Association are the "crème de la crème" of organic agriculture. These foods cannot get certification until the soil has been completely restored and the fruits and vegetables raised in it show certain levels of nutrition in terms of vitamins, minerals, and aminos. They also have excellent taste, high levels of sweetness, and often do not need refrigeration because the level of brix and complex carbohydrates in them preserves them naturally.

The surprising truth is that foods with high levels of minerals and complex carbohydrates in them do not rot when they are not refrigerated. They simply dry out. This is why refrigerators were not really needed until the early part of the 19th century. As soon as we started mass-producing the empty foods of the Modern era, the development of the icebox, and then the refrigerator, was needed to help preserve worthless produce.

When you buy a cucumber and it becomes a pile of slime in the refrigerator within two or three days, you will know it was seriously deficient in minerals. When you buy a bunch of broccoli and find a hollow core going up the stem...when the radishes you slice look like grandmother's lace doilies...if peach pits split open when you try to slice the peach...when strawberries and blueberries are rubbery...when apples are mealy...when lettuce turns to thin, green papery mush...when cauliflower is tough and stringy…when pumpkins, grapefruit, or oranges are spongy or lack juice…these are all foods that are hardly worth the eating because they are seriously deficient in minerals, vitamins, and good nutrition. ❖

Part 3
The Major Detox Routines

14
Introduction to Detox

WHEN WE GET SICK here in America, the first thing we think of is taking some kind of medicine or pill. We focus on putting something *into* the body, usually pills. Seldom do we think of getting well in terms of taking something *out* of the body, like metabolic wastes. The word *detox* means to eliminate something toxic. Although the word was formerly used in terms of alcoholics who went to a hospital to "dry out" or "detox," it has now come to refer to the process of helping people heal by eliminating the waste products that pile up in the body as a result of bad food, sedentary lifestyles, consuming careers, stressful relationships, or other situations in life.

Most of us live in a house or apartment that needs regular cleaning and sometimes a major repair or rebuild. Imagine what it might be like to live in your house for 30 or 40 years and never do the dishes; sweep or vacuum; clean out the closets, the basement, or the garage; replace flooring; or repair the roof.

If brushing your teeth and washing your armpits are equivalent to basic personal housekeeping, most of us could probably say we do a pretty good job of keeping up with our body's personal housekeeping.

Let's say that keeping your colon clean and dissolving plaque in your arteries is equivalent to cleaning out the basement or the garage once or twice a year. How would you rate yourself in this area of personal housekeeping? Do you do this regularly...or do you put it off and just try to get by?

Then, let's say that clearing your liver, lungs, and kidneys of fatty deposits, cellular wastes, and heavy metals is akin to replacing the carpeting, installing a new furnace, and putting on a new roof. Do you attend to these tasks when needed, or do you put them off, sometimes for years, or even sell the house because you don't know how to take care of it?

In a well-known story, the famed Alexis Carrel wanted to find out how long the cells of the body would continue to live and divide because he wanted some clue as to how long the natural, normal, healthy human being should live. He put some cells in a Petri dish, fed them correctly, and rinsed away their waste products every day. To his surprise, they continued to thrive for years. After a while, he realized that it wasn't just the correct nutrition he was providing, it was the fact that he was continually removing their waste products that kept them alive. The experiment only came to an end when Carrel went on a trip and a lab assistant forgot to rinse away the wastes and the cells died.

If you do not take the time to clean and heal your body on a regular basis, you will eventually find you are falling apart as a physical, mental, and emotional system that is unable to maintain any kind of spirit for life. You end up spending your fortune trying to repair the essential parts and systems. Worse, sometimes you discover that they cannot be repaired and you are left with a body you can no longer live in comfortably at all simply because nothing works correctly any more.

There are six major forms of detox: Fasting, the Liver Flush, the Colon Sweep, the Purge, the Castor Oil/Olive Oil Sweat Bath, and the Coffee Enema. [62] Each one does a different kind of clean-up in the body.

Fasting puts the body to rest, lets the immune system focus on fighting bacteria, viruses, and other invaders, allows the body to break down and eliminate widespread, unwanted wastes and tissues, and speeds up repair and rebuilding.

The Liver Flush cleans out the liver, gall bladder, and kidneys and removes plaque from arteries. The Colon Sweep cleans out the small

---

[62] The Liver Flush, Colon Sweep, Purge, Castor Oil/Olive Oil Sweat Bath, and the Coffee Enema are procedures I learned from Dr. Wm. Kelley DDS, and Dr. Nicholas Gonzales MD. Each is a powerful procedure used to heal and restore the body to healthy function.

and large intestines. The Purge alkalinizes the entire body and coaxes cells all over the body to dump their toxic wastes. The Castor Oil/Olive Oil Sweat bath cleans out the skin and the lungs. And the Coffee Enema accomplishes a small daily miracle by forcing the liver to dump its wastes regularly, preventing any toxic build-up. The following chapters describe these and other detox procedures that are extremely powerful in healing our bodies. ❖

15
Fasting

THERE IS AN OLD STORY I've heard several times about a middle-aged man who was not feeling well. He had turned gray, gained a lot of weight, was tired and cranky, argued often with his family and friends, had lost interest in sex, and eventually lost his job. The day he was fired from his job, he went home early and discovered his wife in bed with another man.

This was too much for him, and feeling suicidal, he ran out of the house and into the depths of the forest, abandoning society, his wife, his family and friends, intending to stay in the forest and starve to death.

But as the days without food went by, he began to feel better and better. He lost weight, his energy returned, he felt peaceful inside, and discovered he loved being out in nature. He had accidentally discovered the benefits of fasting.

Eventually, he returned to his village where people were amazed at the trim figure and calm disposition he had developed. He took a new job in a nature sanctuary, found a new, healthy, interesting wife, and spent a long, happy life doing what he loved to do. Every year for the rest of his life he went into the forest, alone and without food, for a period of time. There he renewed himself by fasting.

Hopefully, this little story will help make clear why the most basic rule of thumb in naturopathic healing is: If you get a cold, sinus infection, bronchitis, strep throat, or other problem – STOP EATING UNTIL THE INFECTION CLEARS! The need to digest food creates a huge energy drain on the body, energy that the body should be using to heal itself.

Over the course of any given day or night, your pancreas and entire endocrine system put a great deal of effort into producing enzymes that will *repair* and *rebuild* your physical system. Whenever you eat, your body must temporarily stop producing these repair-and-rebuild enzymes in order to produce *digestive* enzymes. Many foods in their undigested state would be poisonous to the body, so your body breaks these foods down into their most basic components, hoping to extract whatever nutrients might be useful for the ongoing work of repair and rebuilding.

If you don't feel good, the worst thing you can do is eat, especially if you consume sugar or corn syrup. As soon as you eat, you end up feeling worse because the work of healing must be suspended. If you stop eating, your body is free to concentrate on healing and repairing things. In a relatively short time, you'll feel much better.

Well-meaning parents often coax their child to eat when the child doesn't feel good, thus violating the child's natural wisdom, which is to refrain from eating when he's not well. Even animals know better than to eat when they're hurt or sick. They withdraw and sleep, allowing the body to heal itself and not burdening it with the work of digestion.

The unconscious fear that most of us carry is that we will die without food. Although this is true if we are left without food for months, the truth is that we can go quite a long time without something to eat and still do quite well.

One Wednesday night in December, a good friend of mine who lived here on the farm was not feeling well. It was the night of his son's birthday, so in spite of his malaise, he went out to dinner with his boys, where he ate a large prime rib steak, baked potato with all the trimmings, and then birthday cake. Although he felt even worse after this, the next night he went to a party where he again ate and drank heavily, disregarding his body's signals.

By Saturday, he was experiencing severe gastrointestinal cramping and pain that doubled him over every time he tried to eat something. I suggested he stop eating, but he did not seem to hear this and continued to try to eat various things or take medicines he thought might make him feel better. It didn't matter what he tried to take, even a sip of water caused severe cramping that lasted for two or three hours.

Finally, late on Monday night, he asked for a ride to the emergency room of the hospital. He had now been ignoring the signals from his body for five full days and was no longer able to stand the pain. At the hospital the doctors checked him over, looking for anything in terms of obstructed bowel or food poisoning. They ran a few tests, told him they couldn't find anything wrong and said he could go home. He did not feel fine, but he sat up and said, "What should I eat?"

"Eat anything you want," the doctor replied in an unconcerned manner, obviously not understanding that this was not going to work for his distressed patient. My friend and I looked at each other. Until that moment, he wanted to believe that our medical system knew more than his body knew. He was a trained respiratory therapist and very familiar with doctors and hospitals.

On the way home I asked him if he had really considered not eating.

"Don't I need a certain amount of nourishment in order to give my body enough energy to heal?" he asked.

"It *takes* energy to digest food, leaving less energy for healing. You won't die if you stop eating for a while…you'll *heal*. Your body is talking to you. It's telling you it doesn't want to be bothered with food right now," I replied.

When we returned to the farm, I gave him a book to read titled, *Fasting Can Save Your Life*. He read it and was amazed. For eight days, he didn't eat or drink anything except water. On the ninth day, he said, "I think I'm ready to try a little something to eat. What would you recommend?"

I suggested some homemade beef broth since we were in the process of making the potent, highly mineralized broth at that time. Good broth takes three days to make, and there is an old saying that holds much wisdom, "A well-made broth will resurrect the dead." [63] He began with a teaspoonful, increased gradually, and within a few days was eating without pain or difficulty.

I first began personally experimenting with fasting when I was diagnosed with rheumatoid arthritis. Every time I stopped eating, the pain was gone within 24 hours. The problem was that I was already thin

---

[63] Fallon, *Nourishing Traditions,* p. 113.

and couldn't afford to fast for more than ten days at a time. (I'm sure there is a lesson here for all those people who refuse to eat for fear of getting fat. They might think they're nice to look at, but sometimes you need a little reserve weight.) I resolved some of the problem by alternating ten-day periods of detoxification through fasting with ten-day periods of nutrient-dense, easy to digest foods like beef or chicken broth, homemade yogurt, carrot/apple/beet/celery juice, 14-Grain Cereal, or homemade, whole wheat bread with raw butter, and a carefully designed supplement program.

Fasting is so powerful that it's hard to believe it isn't utilized more. When I first began using fasting to heal arthritis, my grand-daughter, Stephanie, was about nine-years-old and subject to constant strep throat and ear infections because of her allergies at that time. One day, my daughter asked me to babysit for Stephie who was home from school with another infection. I had been fasting for three or four days and didn't have the energy to look after a sick child, but I agreed. That morning, I got the idea that maybe Stephie could heal without antibiotics if she fasted as well. I called her mother, a registered nurse, and suggested that Stephie join me in the fast so we could see what would happen. She agreed, and with some caution mixed with adult authority, I explained the situation to my granddaughter.

Being only nine years old, Stephie didn't have much to say and didn't feel good enough to argue. We spent her first day (my fourth day) of fasting by drinking water with a bit of lemon juice in it. The rest of the time we slept. Several times throughout the day, I checked her swollen throat and noted the huge tonsils, which were almost covered with white patches growing on them.

The second day we continued to drink water and rest. Her tonsils were still coated with white, the throat still swollen, and her eyes still droopy and watery looking, but her fever was down a little.

The third day started out much like the first two days. I continued to monitor her condition carefully, aware that I didn't want to be irresponsible with something as serious as a strep infection. I was fully willing to back down and run for antibiotics if she got dramatically worse or if anything really frightening should develop. But around two o'clock that afternoon, when I checked her throat, it was much less swollen, and there were only a few white patches left on her tonsils. I was amazed!

By that evening, her fever was almost gone. She wanted to get up and play, and she began showing an interest in food again. With some difficulty I refused to let her eat, offering only water. We both went to bed early, and the next morning there was a definite improvement.

By noon of the fourth day, the rest of the white patches disappeared from her tonsils, along with the last of her fever. She began asking for something to eat. Uncertain about what to do, but jubilant about the fact that her body had overcome the infection without antibiotics, I continued to insist that she have only water, but promised we would have a little fruit the next morning.

Gradually, offering only fresh, raw fruit and water for two days, then graduating to salads, then her favorite cooked vegetables – potatoes and peas—we returned to eating, adding meat last. That was the last time we ever put any of the children on antibiotics.

Fasting is really quite simple because it requires that you do nothing instead of doing something. You simply stop eating. For the first couple of days, you may be hungry, headachy, and tired. Doing a coffee enema helps these miserable symptoms immensely. By the third day, the hunger stops, and you begin to experience deep changes in your energy system. Often, your inner quiet becomes profound, perception expands, and your physical body starts to relax, slow down, yet heal quickly.

Two things are helpful when you're fasting – the first one is to rest a lot. Don't try to do all the things you normally do. If you must do anything at all, use the time to put together a complete and well-thought-out healing program.

The second thing is a coffee enema once a day for at least the first two or three days to help the liver dump the toxic wastes your body has stored and which the body will immediately begin getting rid of during a fast (see the chapter on *Coffee Enemas*).

Don't be surprised if your skin breaks out, hair seems dull, tongue gets coated, and your breath is awful for a while. These are clear indications that you are getting rid of a lot of inner garbage.

There are many kinds of fasts – water fasts, raw fruit juice fasts, raw vegetable juice fasts, herbal tea fasts, and others. The kind of fast you choose should be somewhat dependent on your goal. Water fasts are fabulous for healing infections or losing weight. Raw fruit juice fasts are powerful for breaking down old, dead, or diseased tissues. Raw vegetable fasts are superb for helping heal after surgery or for building new, healthy cells and tissues. Herbal tea fasts are as varied as the number of herbs on the planet, and each one accomplishes something different. For instance, red clover tea cleans the blood, corn silk tea cleans the bladder, raspberry leaf tea nourishes the reproductive system, and other herbs have other effects, all too numerous to mention here.

Fasting can be practiced for as little as one day, or you can go three days, five days, eight days or more. I have experimented with fasts up to 38 days and found them to be extremely powerful in correcting conditions in the body. When it is time to break the fast, I make a batch of popcorn – no butter or salt – and eat one cup of it slowly, chewing thoroughly. An hour or two later, I eat a second cup, and an hour or two after that, a third cup. This gets the gastrointestinal tract moving nicely again. If you are allergic to popcorn, you could break the fast with oranges or apples, eating two or three of them over a span of 6-8 hours. It is important to re-introduce foods slowly and in small amounts over the first day and not return to eating full meals too quickly.

If you were eating poorly before the fast, do not return to your former diet. Instead, find and incorporate as many real, whole foods into your diet as you can...real milk, butter, eggs, meats, homemade broths and soups, steamed vegetables, breads made with freshly ground whole wheat flour, fresh vegetable juices, and a few good-quality fruits.

If you can get your hands on a book titled *How To Get Well* by Paavo Airola PhD, ND, it is an excellent guide to conducting a variety of juice fasts, among other things. Read *Fasting Can Save Your Life* while you do your first water fast. It is truly an eye opener, and the title says it all. ❖

16
The Liver Flush

WHEN I DEVELOPED rheumatoid arthritis, I became a patient of Dr. Nicholas Gonzales MD in New York, who taught me the great value and power of regular detox in the body. I also followed up my visit to Gonzales with several telephone conversations to Dr. William Kelley, the man who taught Gonzales and who agreed to share what he had learned with me. Although Gonzales has made a few changes to the detox program he teaches, and Kelley insists on a few things of his own, the detox programs that follow in the next three or four chapters are a combination of what they teach, plus what I have learned over the past sixteen years.

There is no organ in the body, with perhaps the exception of the colon, that is as critical as the liver in keeping you healthy and free of toxic waste. When the liver is clogged, you will develop all kinds of problems. These include such things as liver spots, a red nose, intestinal gas, headaches, insomnia, bad breath, poor vision, swollen legs and feet, skin diseases, sterility, appendicitis, allergies, bronchitis, and the more dangerous diseases like cancer, TB, or cirrhosis. Says Raymond Dextreit, "... (you) must realize that there is no cure of any disease, no true health, without a healthy, well-functioning liver." [64]

---

[64] Raymond Dextreit, *Our Earth, Our Cure* (Secaucus, NJ: Carol Publishing Group, translated by Michel Abehsera, 1993) p. 31.

The liver *is* the key to starting any kind of healing, and since the job of the liver is the minute-to-minute detoxification of your entire body, the Liver Flush is an age-old way of making sure this powerful and important organ gets cleaned out and renewed regularly.

To do a Liver Flush you will need:

> 1 gallon of organic apple juice or apple cider
>
> 1 oz of ortho-phosphoric acid (order a 2 oz bottle of *Phosfood* from Standard Process Inc, or *Orthophos* from Nutra-Dyn)
>
> Cal-Amo capsules (from Standard Process)
>
> Epsom salts (from your drug store)
>
> Heavy whipping cream and berries (blueberries or strawberries)
>
> Bentonite liquid (32 oz bottle from Sonné or Progressive Labs)
>
> Olive oil and a fresh lemon

1. **It takes about five days to do a liver flush.** The first four days are fairly simple, but a little planning is required. If you work outside the home, you should plan the start of the liver flush so that you are finishing it on a day when you don't have to go to work the next day. You can work over the first four days, but the fifth day, which is the day of the actual flush, you will want to be at home, at least from 2 pm through the wee hours of the morning. Also, don't schedule your liver flush to end the day before a big party. Party foods and drinks will undo what you just worked so hard to achieve—a clean, unplugged, well-working liver.

2. **To begin:** On the morning of the first day, **add one ounce** (which is 2 TBSP or ½ bottle) of **ortho-phosphoric acid to the gallon of apple juice** and shake well. (Note: you will have to find a chiropractor or nutritional consultant who sells Standard Process or Nutra-Dyn supplements. You can't buy it from a health food store. If all else fails, you can order it from me.) Over the next four to five days, **drink** the entire gallon of apple juice at a rate of **3-4 full (8 oz) glasses a day.** Generally, it takes me four days to drink the majority of the apple juice, with usually 1 or 2 glasses left to be finished on the morning of the fifth day. Drink the juice between meals rather than with meals, and *be sure to brush your teeth with baking soda and rinse your mouth out with soda water after the juice,* using about 1 tsp of soda to a glass of water. This is critical because the two acids in the juice (malic and phosphoric acid) will damage your teeth if you do not use the soda to counteract it. Over

the days that you are drinking the apple juice and phosphoric acid mixture, eat normally.

3. When you begin a liver flush, you should also begin a series of coffee enemas. On each day of the liver flush, **do two coffee enemas** (I call this a "set of coffee enemas") one immediately after the other, **preferably before 7 pm.** Be aware that coffee introduced rectally does not have the same effect as coffee ingested by mouth, and it is not likely to disturb your sleep. However, it's still a good idea to do the coffee enemas in the earlier part of the evening, just in case you're really sensitive to it. The instructions for the coffee enema can be found in a chapter titled *The Coffee Enema,* further along in this book.

4. On the fifth, and last day, of the liver flush, which is the day that you finish the last glass of apple juice, **take 2 capsules of Cal Amo right before breakfast** and take **another 2 capsules right before lunch.** Eat a normal breakfast and lunch on this day, and be sure you finish your lunch by 12 noon. If you are still drinking your apple juice, try to finish the last of it before 2 pm.

5. **At 2 pm, (or 2 hours after your lunch if you've eaten before or after 12 noon), drink 1-2 tablespoons of Epsom salt dissolved in a half-glass of warm water.** You can add a bit of fresh orange, grapefruit, or lemon juice to cover the taste if you like. I follow the Epsom salt drink with a glass of plain water, which is incredibly sweet and delicious after the Epsom salt. After drinking this little concoction, you may want to stay near the bathroom. Your stomach will rumble, your bowels will loosen, and you may or may not have a bowel movement or two.

6. **At 5 pm, or 5 hours after your lunch, again drink 1-2 tablespoons of Epsom salt dissolved in a half glass of warm water.** Add juice if desired, and follow with fresh, cool water. Your intestines will rumble even more, and staying near the bathroom becomes more important!

7. **Between 6–7 pm, or 6 hours after your lunch, take 1 capsule of Cal Amo and eat a dinner that consists of heavy whipping cream and berries.** Any kind of berry is acceptable, but it's the cream that is important, so eat as much as you want. I put frozen blueberries in a cereal bowl and pour a cup of the cream over them. Usually, I eat two bowls of this delicious mixture. You can also put the blueberries and cream in a blender to make a blended shake, just be careful not to leave

the blender on too long or you'll have butter instead of cream with your blueberries.

8. **At 10:30 pm, (or ½ hour before you go to bed) drink ¼ cup of Bentonite liquid**, which is actually clay in a liquid suspension. It doesn't taste bad, in fact, it doesn't have any taste, just a creamy texture, but it performs small miracles in your intestinal tract. It attracts to itself both parasites and the silty, toxic wastes dumped by the liver, helping to carry these out of the body later.

9. **One-half hour later, at 11 pm, (and just before going to bed) drink ½ cup of olive oil.** The juice of one fresh lemon can be added to the olive oil, and this makes it much more palatable. We squeeze the lemon juice into the olive oil, shake vigorously or blend briefly with a stick blender, and put it in the freezer for 15-20 minutes. This is much easier to drink than straight olive oil! It may take you 10-15 minutes or so to drink the entire ½ cup, but immediately after finishing the oil, **go to bed and lie down on your right side with knees drawn up. Stay in that position for at least 30 minutes**. You might even fall asleep and stay in that position for a couple of hours, which is all right.

10. Between 1-3 am, the liver enters its most active period of the day, and you may waken feeling nauseated. This is because of the release of stored toxins from the gallbladder and the liver. If you are quite toxic, you might experience more than a little nausea. You may vomit, have diarrhea, or a serious "night sweat" alternating with chills. *To avoid all this, get up about 1:30 am and do a set of coffee enemas.* This not only aids the liver in dumping even more of its toxins, it helps move them out of the body before they can make you sick. In actuality, it is a very good sign if you feel nauseous or have other symptoms of toxicity because it means that the liver and gallbladder are actually flushing themselves out and the healing procedure is working. When you have finished the set of coffee enemas, go back to bed and to sleep for the rest of the night.

11. **The next day, eat normally and take two (2) Cal Amo with breakfast, two (2) Cal Amo with lunch, and one (1) Cal Amo with dinner**. You may feel a little low the next day, although many people have no aftereffects at all.

❖

Now, what is this procedure about, and why do you need each step? A simpler version of the liver flush was first used during the 1920s as a way of improving liver function. The procedure outlined above is an improvement and refinement of the original technique and serves the healing process in several important ways.

First, when you put the ortho-phosphoric acid into the apple juice, you now have a drink containing two acids: the malic acid that is found naturally in apple juice, and the phosphoric acid that you added. These two acids work together to dissolve plaque, calcium deposits, and other "stony" deposits in the arteries, liver, and elsewhere. They soften and dissolve gallstones and kidney stones, reducing them to sand and gravel.

There are two kinds of aging. One is chronological aging, the other is biological aging. One of the criteria for determining your biological age has to do with how soft, flexible, and deposit-free your organs and tissues are. Some authorities consider aging to be due simply to hardening, also known as *sclerosis*, of the body tissues. A baby's tissues and organs are soft, pliable, and free of waste deposits, which is why they often have such good health. By removing sclerotic material in your body, you free your arteries and organs to work better and reverse your biological age.

Drinking the apple juice with its two acids over the course of five days dissolves a lot of this sclerotic matter. The liver then filters this toxic material out of your blood, and the liver flush then flushes it out of your body altogether.

On the day of the actual flush, the two doses of Epsom salt, which contains high levels of magnesium, relax the openings of the gallbladder and the bile ducts. Ordinarily, the mouth of the gallbladder is like a set of tight, firm, rosebud-like lips with a very tough, small opening. When you drink the Epsom salts, those tightly pursed lips relax, soften, and open.

Then, along comes a good dose of cream with a few berries in it! And what happens to the liver and gallbladder? The job of these two organs is to emulsify fat, and cream is pure fat. So the liver and gallbladder immediately and vigorously contract, squirting bile onto the cream—along with the softened, shrunken gallstones, stored wastes in the liver, and any sand- or gravel-like material that has accumulated in them. All of this passes easily into the small intestine, which is why you may waken in the night feeling nauseous.

The clay you drink around 10:30 pm not only helps to bulk up the wastes so you can excrete them more easily, it is a powerful healing agent in its own right, as is the olive oil, which is a specific healing agent for mucous membranes and tissues in the digestive tract.

Be aware that each step in the liver flush performs a key role in the sequence of events that lead to a clean, healthy liver. Do not skip any of the steps or try to substitute procedures or you will not get the results you are working for.

All in all, the liver flush is a simple yet powerful way of removing gallstones without surgery, cleaning out your liver, removing plaque from arteries and organs, eliminating hot flashes and insomnia, improving eyesight, lifting depression, eliminating the effects of chemotherapy, and dispelling numerous other problems while improving function throughout the body. Since the liver is the organ that produces your cholesterol, a liver flush also helps to normalize cholesterol metabolism. I have had people tell me that the liver flush dropped their cholesterol level by 35 points almost overnight.

A number of people have asked if they can do a liver flush when they don't have a gall bladder or perhaps have had a colostomy. The answer is "yes" in both cases.

An even greater number of people have also asked about doing a liver flush while undergoing chemotherapy. Perhaps sharing a story will answer this best. About a year and a half ago, a woman named Kristin had just had surgery for colon cancer and was undergoing chemo. She heard about these healing methods from a friend and called to register for one of my classes. On the day of class, she arrived, terribly thin, with huge dark circles under her eyes, tired, and adamant about not putting her body through any more difficulty. For the entire weekend, she listened carefully, asked really tough questions, and left at the end of the weekend still uncertain as to whether or not she should try the liver flush, especially since she was in the middle of chemo. I had encouraged her tentatively, based on the reports from other people who had done remarkably well after starting detox while in chemotherapy, yet I felt this was a decision she had to make for herself. A few days later she returned to buy the few specialty things she needed, then went home to start.

A week later I answered the phone to find an ecstatic voice on the other end of the line. It was Kristin. She had finished the liver flush a day or two earlier and said, "I can't believe the difference in how I feel. It's like a black, oppressive cloud has been lifted from my mind, my heart, and my body!" She went on for a few minutes, excitedly sharing how glad she was to have done the liver flush, about how uncertain she

had been because she'd already been through so much, and what a
wondrous sense of life and good feeling now filled her.

Others have shared similar things, whether they were healing
from cancer, dieting to lose weight, struggling with congestive heart
failure, or trying to recover from some other illness. The liver flush is
meant to be used about three times a year, an average of once every
fourth month (e.g. January, May, and September). Get a calendar, mark
off the five days needed to complete this detox procedure, then keep that
date with yourself and your health. If you do, you will be amazed at the
results. You will look and feel younger and will keep your body in good
working order. ❖

17
The Colon Sweep

WHEN YOUR SMALL INTESTINE starts to plug up with waste matter, it doesn't necessarily become blocked in the sense that nothing will pass through it. Rather, it becomes so clogged with a thick layer of gunk that the cilia in the intestine no longer work well. Intestinal cilia are thin, filament-like fingers that line the inside walls of the intestine. When clean and healthy, they wave back and forth like grasses in the wind, filtering the remains of food through their fine fingers while extracting and absorbing the vitamins, minerals, enzymes, and other nutrients that pass over their surfaces.

As these cilia become clogged with layers of thick, sticky wastes, your ability to absorb the nutrients needed to constantly rebuild and repair your body goes – no pun intended – right down the tubes.

The large intestine, also known as the colon, is a long tube that begins in the lower right quadrant of the abdomen and rises upward (the ascending colon) to about your waistline where it makes a 90° turn and goes across the abdomen (the transverse colon) to the left side of your body. From there, it slants upward, passing under the left ribs, then down (the descending colon) in an S-shaped fashion to the rectum.

Over time, the inside of the colon begins to build up a layer of gunk that tends to have a paralyzing effect on the ability of the colon to move, thus bowel movements slow down, get farther apart, and not all the waste matter is removed. This thick, gunky layer is also a good place for bacteria to make their home, and as these bacteria multiply and leave their own wastes, the colon can go from irritation to inflammation to a state known as "leaky gut syndrome." This is a condition in which the tissue of the colon is so weakened, it begins to allow waste matter to leak into the body, poisoning you and causing all manner of havoc. This seriously drains the resources of the immune system, which struggles to deactivate the constant invasions of bacteria and other toxic materials coming through the wall of the colon into the sensitive areas of the abdomen.

For a moment now, picture the transverse colon like a rope bridge suspended across a chasm. Then, imagine that someone comes along and starts loading boxes onto the bridge. It may hold up well for a while, but as the load gets heavier, the bridge starts to droop seriously.

The same thing happens with the colon. As the layer of gunk in the colon thickens, the transverse colon gets heavier and heavier. It can end up drooping so far down into the abdomen in a "U-shape" that it lays on top of other organs, interfering with their functions. Intestines, bladder, sexual organs, and rectum can all have great difficulty going about their daily business with the heavy colon sitting on top of them.

Worse, as the heavily stuffed colon stretches and droops, it ceases to work effectively at all and constipation sets in. Food goes in, drops to the bottom of the loop, and the colon is neither strong enough nor flexible enough to push it back up and on out. As waste backs up in the system, pockets can bulge out here and there, creating perfect breeding places for infection. Meanwhile, your eyesight gets worse, skin looks terrible, hair falls out, breath gets bad, joints get stiffer, and you succumb to every cold and flu or other infection that comes around. Thus, cleaning the colon on a regular basis is equally as important as flushing your liver.

More than once I have heard the old saying, "Death begins in the colon." If either the colon or small intestine begins to plug up with old waste matter, elimination backs up and absorption of nutrients slows down. I know people who only have a bowel movement every four or five days. A healthy colon will expel some matter after every meal. If you eat three times a day, that would amount to three bowel movements a day.

To do a Colon Sweep you will need:

> 1 gallon of organic apple juice
>
> 1 bottle of Intestinal Bulking Agent II (available from Holistic Horizons)

4-5 qts of yogurt containing live cultures (Do not use any low fat yogurts.)

1 bottle of Acidophilus with capsules containing at least 4-5 billion live cultures per capsule; preferably a probiotic with 10 billion live organisms per dose

1. **It takes ten days to complete the full Colon Sweep**. You may eat your normal meals during the colon sweep, and if you work outside the home you can continue to go to work. However, plan to start your Colon Sweep on a Friday or Saturday because the first day or two, there is often a heavy, crampy feeling in the gut and sometimes a nagging headache.

2. **At 10 am,** or sometime halfway between breakfast and lunch, put **8 oz of organic apple juice in a shaker** cup or mason jar that has a lid. **Add 1 rounded tsp of Intestinal Bulking Agent II** to the juice, cover and **shake vigorously** to mix well, then **drink immediately**. If you let it sit for even a few minutes, it begins turning to jelly due to the pectin in the Bulking Agent.

3. **Immediately after drinking the juice and bulking agent, drink 8 oz of water**, downing it completely. You may feel a bit full after this, which is normal.

4. **At 3 pm, or halfway between lunch and supper, repeat Steps 2 and 3**, taking a second dose of bulking agent in apple juice, and following this immediately with 8 oz of water.

5. **At 8 pm, or halfway between supper and bedtime, repeat Steps 2 and 3**, taking your third dose of bulking agent and again following with 8 oz of water.

6. Sometime **between 3 pm and 8 pm, do a set of two coffee enemas,** one immediately after the other.

7. **Eat ½ cup of yogurt at bedtime.**

8. **Repeat Steps 2 through 7 each day for five days until you have taken a total of fifteen (15) doses of Bulking Agent.** This completes part one of the Colon Sweep.

9. **For the next five days** the procedure consists of the critical step of replenishing your bacterial flora. **Eat ½ cup of yogurt with each meal, and take two Acidophilus capsules with warm water on an empty stomach at bedtime. Sprinkle a dose of probiotic powder on your normal meals—breakfast, lunch, and dinner.**

❖

What was happening during the colon sweep, and why do you do this detox procedure? First, the bulking agent can absorb many times its own weight in water and enlarges in much the same way as a sponge does when exposed to water. As mentioned above, you may feel discomfort the first day or two due to the expansion of the bulking agent in the intestinal tract. The discomfort is a good sign because it means the bulking agent is stretching the intestines to maximum diameter.

This swollen mass then begins working its way through the small and large intestines, filling every nook and cranny, scrubbing, scraping, and forcing out all manner of stored wastes that would not otherwise be excreted.

Most people doing the colon sweep will pass a variety of exotic particles and substances. Many describe passing long casings, similar to a snakeskin or sausage casing, which is actually the dried mucus and dead cells from the surface of the intestines and colon. These wastes accumulate over a period of many years and seriously interfere with the absorption of nutrients and your ability to expel waste.

This procedure is also the most effective way of removing abnormal bacteria and other organisms from the gut that take hold after antibiotics have been used. These harmful organisms and bacteria are scraped away, but so are the beneficial organisms, and it is for this reason that the yogurt and acidophilus are so essential. After a colon sweep, candida albicans, staph, strep, and other virulent organisms that live in your gastrointestinal tract and whose job it is to finish breaking down the food you have eaten, will grow quickly and replace themselves in short order. The beneficial organisms that control these more virulent bacteria are much slower to grow. If you do not eat the yogurt and take the acidophilus for *at least five days*, you can end up with severe gastritis, candida, bloating, gas, and other difficulties related to food and digestion. Save yourself the trouble, and if you are going to err, err on the side of a few *extra* days of yogurt, not a few less.

❖

Once you have completed the Liver Flush and the Colon Sweep, you are half way through the first round of detox procedures. At this point, I often hear things like, "I haven't had a single migraine or even a headache...The flu skipped over me this year...I didn't realize how bloated I was until after that Colon Sweep, and I had to hitch my belt a notch tighter...It seems impossible, but I think my eyesight has improved...There's still a little stiffness in the morning, but I could swear my arthritis pain has almost disappeared...Even though the weather is cold, I haven't had my usual difficulties breathing..." and other reports of improved function.

At this point in the program, there is a jump in your body's ability to absorb the nutrition in the foods you're eating and the supplements you're taking, and many people begin healing rapidly. This is a critical step in healing because you can put all the good food and medicine in the world into your system, but if it passes through unabsorbed, you won't heal. Sometimes people only notice a slight lessening of the problem that was bothering them at this point, but those who continue to detoxify themselves notice steady improvement in every area of life, health, and energy, as well as the function of the entire body/mind system.

This improvement makes it easier to keep going, so let's move on to the next step in the full detox program, the Purge. ❖

18
The Purge

THE PURGE IS ONE of the most important detox routines, especially for those with infections or those who have cancers. Several versions of the technique exist, but the best one is outlined in the original edition of Dr. William Kelley's book, *One Answer To Cancer*. [65]

William D. Kelley DDS, cured himself of pancreatic cancer when he was in his late 30s by refusing to give in to the disease. By understanding nutrition and by developing a series of detox routines designed to clean out the toxic by-products of disease, he was able to support the life processes in his body until full healing occurred. In Kelley's view, the Purge is the most powerful of the detox procedures because it puts the body at rest, which aids the rapid removal of metabolic wastes. In addition, the purge pushes the body into an alkaline state in which repair and rebuilding of damaged tissues occurs rapidly.

In Kelley's view, people who develop cancers are not doomed to death at all, because it is relatively simple to stop these growths and even their metastases, but it is much trickier to get the body to break down and remove dead cancer tissue. This dead tissue is extremely poisonous and more often than not, it is this poisonous run-off that kills the individual

---

[65] Kelley's book, *One Answer to Cancer*, is available on the Internet. Simply type the name of the book into Google or your search engine and it will come up. I use – **www.whale.to/a/kelley**.html.

by plugging up the liver, lungs, skin, and kidneys, clouding the brain's orders, messing up endocrine function, impeding digestion and half a dozen other bodily activities, and generally making you so sick that you don't care if you live or die. Of course, as soon as you get to that point, your cells know you have given up, and they give up. You become history.

Although the poisonous run-off from asthma, diabetes, or arthritis isn't quite as powerful as that from cancer, there is a continuous accumulation of wastes from these diseases. In addition, poorly built and poorly functioning tissues and cells within the main systems of the body also need to be cleared out regularly. If you do not clear toxic debris from your body, you will have great difficulty healing and may only get worse. Thus, the value of the Purge is in its power to remove large amounts of waste from the body, including waste material from *inside* your cells, in a quick and efficient manner.

To do The Purge you will need:

> Plenty of fresh fruit and salad fixings
>
> A juicing machine or hand reamer for citrus fruits
>
> 12 grapefruits
>
> 12 lemons
>
> 24 oranges
>
> 1-gallon jug or pitcher
>
> Epsom Salt (from your local drug store)
>
> 1 gallon of distilled or purified water (from your local grocery store and sometimes known as Reverse Osmosis or R.O. water)
>
> Cal-Amo capsules (from Standard Process)
>
> Yogurt

It takes five days to complete the medium-length version of the Purge, and if you work outside the home, you can continue to work for the first two days. The next two days you will have to be at home and near the bathroom, so plan to start your Purge on a Thursday and Friday so you can be at home on Saturday and Sunday. The last day of the Purge is similar to the first two days, so you can go back to work without difficulty.

Days 1 & 2

Days 1 and 2 of the Purge are fairly simple and normal. They consist of eating only **fresh fruit for breakfast and through the morning, a large salad full of raw vegetables for lunch and dinner on both days, and doing a set of coffee enemas in the late afternoon or early evening**. Eating fresh fruit does not mean you eat an apple or a banana and then starve the rest of the morning. It means eating until you are satisfied. If that means two bananas, a kiwi, an apple, and a bowl of strawberries over the course of the morning, then that is what you need to have on hand.

A salad for lunch and dinner does not mean three pieces of iceberg lettuce, with one wedge of tomato and two slices of cucumber. It means a big salad of mixed greens, chopped tomatoes, fresh parsley, cucumbers, carrots, cabbage, radishes, peas, kohlrabi, green beans, broccoli, cauliflower, and finely diced onion, sprinkled with garlic salt and black pepper, and generous doses of virgin olive oil, melted butter, and flaxseed oil mixed with the juice of a fresh lemon drizzled over the top.

I use 2 TBSP olive oil mixed with 2 TBSP melted butter (not margarine) and 2 TBSP flaxseed oil with the juice of ½ lemon. For variation, add up to 1 TBSP of dried or 2 TBSP of fresh herbs such as oregano and basil, or parsley and savory, or dill and thyme. Make the dressing early, then leave it in the refrigerator overnight to release the herb flavors. If the butter hardens in the refrigerator, do NOT warm the dressing in the microwave to melt it again. In fact, never use a microwave for anything because it so completely deranges the frequencies in the molecules of the food that they become destructive to you instead of nourishing you. Just warm the container briefly in a bowl of warm water. Or, put all the ingredients together except for the butter and flaxseed oil, adding them just before serving.

When I am eating only salad, I start by filling a 1 QT bowl, eat it all, and sometimes refill it. If I get hungry in mid-afternoon, I have another bowl-full. You will find you can eat a lot of salad without feeling stuffed. The biggest problem I run into is all the chewing required. I get tired of chewing, yet it's very important to chew the raw foods in your salad very well. Do not eat after 8 pm. If you get hungry, drink a pint of water, then try meditating, doing some gentle stretching exercises, or go to bed early and sleep so you won't know you're hungry. If you're desperately hungry, eat an apple.

Day 3

1. On the morning of Day 3, **arise about 6:30 am** and dissolve 1 TBSP of Epsom salt in a half-glass of distilled or Reverse Osmosis (R.O.) water, stirring until completely dissolved. **Drink this combination of Epsom salt and water**, following it with a half-glass of plain or purified water, which will taste delicious after the Epsom salt!

2. **At 7 am**, which is one-half hour later, **take another tablespoon of Epsom salt dissolved in a half-glass of R.O. water**, followed by a half-glass of plain or purified water.

3. **At 7:30 am**, which is one-half hour later, **take a third tablespoon of Epsom salt dissolved in a half-glass of R.O. water**, followed by a half-glass of plain or purified water. You will now have taken three doses of Epsom salt over a 1 hour period.

4. **Next, make a citrus punch** consisting of the following:

Juice of 6 grapefruits

Juice of 6 lemons

Juice of 12 oranges

Put all the juice from the above fruits into a gallon jug. When finished juicing, you should have between ½ and ¾ of a gallon of juice. Then add distilled or Reverse Osmosis water until the gallon jug is full. You now have 1 gallon of "citrus punch." It takes about an hour to make the citrus punch, so don't wait until it's time to drink the first glass to start making it; plan accordingly.

5. **Approximately two hours after the last dose of Epsom salt, (about 9:30 am) drink an 8-10 oz glass of this citrus punch.**

6. Thereafter, **drink a glass of the punch every hour.** You are to **eat no food that day** except, if you wish, an orange for dinner.

7. With your **12:30 pm glass of punch**, take **1 capsule of Cal Amo**.

8. With your **6:30 pm glass of punch**, take a **2nd capsule of Cal Amo**.

9. With your **10:30 pm glass of punch**, take a **3rd capsule of Cal Amo**.

10. **Finish drinking the entire gallon of citrus punch in one day.** During the purge, you may feel a variety of symptoms, such as nausea, headaches, muscle aches, and pains. Such symptoms indicate the body is releasing stored wastes, and although you might be uncom-

fortable, do not be alarmed. If you become seriously nauseous or have a very bad headache, do a set of coffee enemas in the afternoon. If necessary, do another set at night. **Rest a lot during the day.** Stay close to the bathroom.

Day 4

On Day 4, **repeat the entire set of instructions for Day 3,** including the three doses of Epsom salt, drinking the gallon of citrus punch made from grapefruit, lemons, and oranges, and taking the Cal Amo. You can expect to spend a lot of time running to the bathroom again. You will also notice that what's coming out looks just like what's going in! Dr. Kelley recommends that if you have cancer, you repeat the Epsom Salt and citrus punch routine for a third day, extending the Purge for an extra day because it is so good at removing wastes. He mentions that for every gallon of the citrus punch you drink, an equivalent gallon of waste material is removed from body cells and tissues. That's a lot of waste!

Day 5

On Day 5, (or Day 6, if you extended the Purge an extra day) return to the fresh fruit and salads that were eaten on Day 1 and Day 2. At each meal on Day 5, include ½ cup of Yogurt. Do a set of coffee enemas in the late afternoon or early evening. After that, you can return to your everyday food, routines, and supplements until the next round of detox.

❖

As mentioned above, the power of the Purge is in its ability to soften cell walls and allow removal of stored wastes, toxins, and other useless material from the cells and tissues of the body.

It bears repeating that the Liver Flush cleans the liver, gall bladder, kidneys, and cardiovascular system by removing stony material, fatty deposits, plaque, the remains of old chemicals picked up by the liver, and sometimes even bone spurs from your system. These things may not be immediately life threatening, but they interfere with your body's efforts to maintain itself and keep working in a normal way.

The Colon Sweep is used to clear gunky material in both the small intestine and large intestine. In doing so, it forces a rebuilding of the absorptive surfaces in the small intestine, which then greatly improves your ability to absorb the nutrition needed for healing. And the material is clears from the large intestine brings biochemical changes that benefit the entire body.

You use the Purge when you need to clean out tissues in the rest of the body that the Liver Flush and Colon Sweep do not specifically reach. Use the Purge to help break down and eliminate cancers, mucous in the lungs, waste material in the skin, and useless, interfering waste products everywhere. The Purge is so powerful that I have seen it do away with the beginning signs of cervical cancer or cancer of the eye with just one 3-day Purge.

The Liver Flush, Colon Sweep, and Purge are like tools in your healing toolbox, meant to be used to accomplish certain goals. Hopefully, at this point, you are beginning to get a feel for these healing tools and how or when to use them.

Only a few examples of when to use these three forms of detox might include…using the Liver Flush to get relief from hot flashes. The Colon Sweep is useful for scrubbing the colon and removing small growths and polyps, or clearing away Candida while the yogurt/ acidophilus regimen re-establishes the correct balance of micro-organisms in the gut. The Purge is extremely good at clearing up lingering bronchitis or pneumonia. In years past, before surgery became big business, the Liver Flush was used to remove gallstones and improve digestion. And I think I've already said that the Purge is excellent in clearing the effects of chemotherapy.

Although there are other forms of detox that we will cover next, these three procedures are the basic tools needed to keep the body clean, youthful, and functioning in a healthy fashion. ❖

19
Castor Oil/Olive Oil Sweat Bath

THE BODY USES FOUR main systems to excrete waste materials: the liver and gastrointestinal tract, the kidneys, the lungs, and the skin. Too often, we forget that the skin can be used to help seriously detoxify the body and speed the removal of metabolic wastes.

If you begin using the program outlined in this book, or even just change your diet to include more whole, healthy foods, the body will begin taking advantage of these and will make an effort to repair and rebuild itself even more vigorously. As it does so, it will break down old, poorly-built cells and begin mobilizing stored wastes to be removed. The toxic run-off from the breakdown of metabolic debris, and especially that from cancers or other illnesses, tends to accumulate too rapidly for the body to excrete through its main channels, and the result can be all sorts of skin eruptions and blemishes from pimples to liver spots, from rashes to open sores. Such conditions may be worrisome, but should be viewed as a sign that it's time to do a castor oil/olive oil sweat bath.

When I started regular detox after visiting Dr. Gonzales, my skin began to break out with a dark red, terribly itchy rash. My forehead, eyelids, breastbone, shin bones, and forearms were the places most affected. My eyelids became so swollen that the lid over my right eye split in two places. When I called Gonzales, he told me to "...tough it out!" and asked if I was doing the sweat baths. When I said no, he suggested I start them immediately. I should have listened, but I didn't, and I was sorry. Even though the eyelid healed without trouble, I continued to suffer from an ugly rash with an itch that drove me crazy for another four months.

When I finally found time to do the castor oil/olive oil sweat baths, they turned out to be almost miraculous in their ability to clear up skin.

To do a Castor Oil/Olive Oil Sweat Bath you will need:

2 TBSP castor oil (cold-pressed and organic)

2 TBSP olive oil (extra virgin, cold pressed, organic)

A bathtub with a slip-proof mat in the bottom

1 QT of purified or R.O. (reverse osmosis) water and cup or glass

1 t-shirt, a sweat shirt, a pair of sweat pants, and heavy socks

Several large bath towels

Oatmeal or glycerin soap (no deodorant soaps, please)

A bed with 3-4 heavy blankets or quilts

A rubber sheet, old shower curtain, or piece of plastic (optional)

1. **It takes about one morning to do a sweat bath**. You can also do the sweat bath in the evening if you prefer. Total time is about 2-3 hours. If you do the sweat bath in the morning, **do not eat any breakfast beforehand**. If you do one in the evening, skip supper so that you have an empty stomach. If you are going to do one in the afternoon and you have eaten lunch, wait at least three hours. Your body should not be burdened with the job of trying to digest food when you are asking it to dump toxins. You will be *much more uncomfortable* if you have just eaten a meal. You can get something light to eat afterwards even if it's late at night. And you may feel so wonderful that you might not want to eat anything for a few hours afterwards, since food is a serious disturbance in the body.

2. Let's assume you are going to do your sweat bath in the morning. **When you get up in the morning, brush your teeth with a non-fluoride toothpaste. Drink one cup of purified or R.O. water.**

3. **Prepare your bed** by laying a piece of plastic, a rubber sheet, or an old, plastic shower curtain over the pillow and fitted sheet that covers your mattress and mattress pad. This will keep them from getting wet and sweat-stained. Double up one towel and put it over the pillow. Put two heavy towels where you will lay down and sweat. Try to position the towels so that they will catch most of the sweat from your body. Get

out extra quilts or blankets and put them nearby so you can cover up with them when you lay down to sweat.

4. **In a small bowl, mix 2 TBSP of castor oil with 2 TBSP of olive oil, stirring well**. Take this mixture to your bathroom, along with the t-shirt, sweatshirt, sweat pants, heavy socks, another couple of towels, the quart of purified water, and the cup or glass. Put the drinking water and the cup on the edge of the tub or someplace where you can easily reach it once you are in the tub.

5. **Turn on the hot water in the tub and begin filling it with water as hot as you can stand it and as deep as you can make it**. If your hot water heater is small and you don't think you will have enough to fill the tub, you may want to heat some water in a large pot on the stove and add it to the tub, then add water from the tap to get as much hot water as possible. The shallower the water, the faster it will cool, and you need it to stay hot enough long enough to get yourself into a good sweat. Just don't burn yourself. We usually make sure the water is at least 108-110°. If it's less, you may have to sit longer and add more hot water after 10-15 minutes in order to get the body up to temperature.

6. While the tub is filling, **get completely undressed, and rub the oil mixture into your skin from head to toe**. If you have long hair, tie your hair up on *top* of your head and out of the way. Make sure that you do not have a ponytail or knot of hair at the *back* of your head that will make it uncomfortable for you to lie back in the tub or in the bed once you get to the sweating portion of the routine. You can rub some of the oil into your hairline about an inch or so, and if you wish, you can also massage a little into your scalp by dipping just your fingertips lightly into the oil then doing a fingertip massage of the scalp, but do not saturate your hair. And *do not put oil on the soles of your feet* or they'll be too slippery when you're stepping into and out of the tub.

7. When the tub is full, and with the oil now spread over your body, **get into the tub and soak in the hot water**. Be careful getting into the tub as you will be quite slippery! Once in, try to lie back so that everything but your face is under water. If necessary, turn over onto your stomach for five minutes, sticking your legs up out of the water to get the trunk of your body into the hot water. Sit up again once you start to sweat. Take a clock or wristwatch with you and **stay in the hot water for 15-25 minutes, or until you are sweating profusely.** If the water is shallow and starts to cool off, let a little bit of it out and put some fresh hot water in.

If you are really sick or weakened, it's a good idea to **have someone around to keep an eye and an ear out for you.** Ask them to come to the bathroom door once or twice during the soaking period and ask, "Are you doing okay in there?" If you need help, say so. If you live alone, ask a friend to come over and just read or have a cup of tea nearby while you're doing the sweat bath. If, by chance, you should become faint, or slip and fall, you'll have someone to help you.

If the water is nice and hot, you will usually start to be uncomfortably warm after about five minutes. The tendency is to hold your breath, but don't do this. Don't breathe in extra-deep gulps either. Breathe steadily, easily, and in a relaxed manner. You will feel most uncomfortable just before the body breaks into a sweat. **Once you start to sweat, begin drinking water from the quart of purified R.O. water** you brought to the tub. Keep sipping at the water as you sweat. Drinking not only replaces the water you're losing through sweat, it gives you something to do when you're so hot, sweaty, and uncomfortable.

The hot bath allows the oils to penetrate to the deepest levels of the skin, and both the castor oil and the olive oil are nutrients as well as healers of skin and mucous membranes.

I usually tell people that, once I get in the tub, I stay until I get to the point that I think I'm going to melt or pass out, then stay for five minutes longer!

Once your heart is going at a very good clip in its efforts to cool down the body, you are ready to get out of the tub.

8. **When it is time to get out of the tub**, pull the plug to let the water out and climb out of the tub but *do not stand up straight. Stay bent at the waist to keep your head about level with your hips.* If you try to stand up, you may find you are too light-headed. Again, be careful getting out of the tub because you will be quite slippery. **You should also be sweating heavily, breathing fast, and have a pounding heart.** Take a towel, sit on the toilet seat cover or a nearby chair, and quickly dry yourself as much as possible, which will be difficult because of the continuous sweat.

9. **Immediately put on the heavy socks, t-shirt, sweatshirt, and sweat pants. Wrap the towel around your head.**

10. **Get into your bed and cover up with the sheet, blanket, and at least two quilts.** Pull the covers right up to the bottom of your nose to keep you hot and sweating as long as possible. Stay under the covers for one hour. During this time you will feel like you have become

one giant, beating heart, and you will sweat prodigiously. This sweating stimulates the release of poisons and toxic waste matter through your skin. It also has an extraordinary effect on the lungs, clearing them dramatically.

11. After about half an hour or so, you will notice that your heart is slower, you are cooling down a bit, and the sweating is beginning to slow up. If you are drowsy, drift off into a little nap. This will be wonderfully healing for you. **When an hour has gone by, or when you wake up, your heart should be quiet, your breath should be normal, and you, as well as everything around you, should be soaking wet.** At this point, the sweating portion is done.

12. **Get up, peel off the wet clothing (you *will* be soaked through), and go take a *warm* shower using an oatmeal or a glycerin soap** both of which are gentle on skin. Try not to use the commercial soaps you see advertised on television as they are often quite harsh and contain chemicals that are difficult for the skin to handle. Wash and condition your hair as usual. And be careful getting in and out of the shower if that shower is also the bathtub you were soaking in earlier. It may have a thin film of oil in it!

13. **When you get out of the shower, get a clean, dry towel and begin drying yourself off with a *slow*, pressured motion that removes dead skin. Sometimes the dead skin on your arms and legs comes off in thousands of tiny rolls**. Continue removing dead skin until the new skin underneath is bright pink, soft, and glowing. If an area of skin dries before you have a chance to rub it with the towel, dampen the skin with warm water for a few minutes or so, then continue rubbing briskly.

14. When you are done rubbing dead skin from every area of your body you can reach, **get dressed in clean, preferably cotton clothing. Do not put any creams, oils, or lotions on your skin for 24 hours**. Leave it clean and clear to breathe easily, without the impediment of lotions and potions.

15. **Strip the bed of its wet sheets. Throw these into the washer and then the dryer, along with your wet clothes and towels,** and you are finished.

❖

When you have completed the entire sweat bath routine, you will notice a distinct difference in the depth, clarity, and ease of your breathing. Not only does it feel like you are breathing easily all the way through your chest, this feeling extends down into the abdomen! It's almost as if every organ and system in the trunk of the body has been turned into a set of lungs. It can also feel as if you are breathing right through your skin, and there is an unusual sense of being alive that has to be experienced in order to be understood.

After 24 hours, you may take a *warm* shower using a washcloth or back brush to rub the body briskly but without soap. Let the water run over your skin as long as you can. Afterward, massage in a thin coating of a good, herbal oil or moisturizing lotion. You will be surprised at how beautiful, flexible, and healthy your skin looks, even after 24 hours with no lotions! You will realize that your skin becomes old-looking, dry, wrinkled, and sallow because you haven't bothered to clean it well and a thick layer of dead cells has built up on the surface.

The castor oil/olive oil sweat bath is one of the most valuable of the detox routines and is a potent restorative. This is especially true for someone who has cancer, lung disease, or one of the forms of arthritis. As a side note…if you have cancer, don't be surprised if the water in the tub turns brownish or blackish after you've been sweating a bit. This just means you are getting rid of a lot of toxins.

In a full detox program the **castor oil/olive oil sweat bath should be done once a week for 12 weeks** in the first three months of the program. After that they can be discontinued until the following year when they should be repeated.

I live in Michigan and have found that it is best to do the sweat bath series each year from mid-December through mid-March. This is the coldest time of the year and the sweat baths are a wonderful way to ward off lung congestion, head colds, sinus infections, and the stiffness that generally accompanies cold weather. You can certainly start them at any other time of the year if you have contracted a catastrophic illness and need to implement a full detox program, but for annual maintenance the winter months are a great time to do them.

Don't hesitate to do a sweat bath if you should get the flu, catch a cold, or develop any other temporary problem. They are wonderful for healing almost everything. ❖

20
The Coffee Enema

THE COFFEE ENEMA HAS been used for over 100 years as a generalized detox procedure and was once listed in the Merck Manual as a powerful detoxifying and healing practice. Despite rumors to the contrary, coffee enemas are perfectly safe when you follow the guidelines. Coffee enemas stimulate the liver and gallbladder to release stored toxins and wastes, and this improves and enhances liver function. When Dr. Nicholas Gonzales inquired as to why coffee enemas were removed from the Merck Manual, he was told that it was considered "too old-fashioned."

To do a Coffee Enema you will need:

A stainless steel or glass coffee maker, drip style is fine.

1 QT plus ¼ cup of distilled, or R.O. water, or spring water

2 TBSP of organic coffee (no decaf)

1 disposable enema bag (can be re-used many times)

KY jelly (or wheat germ oil, olive oil, Vitamin E oil)

A hook on the wall to hang the bag from, or a hanger to hang the enema bag from the shower curtain rod.

1 rubber colon tube (optional)

1 TBSP unsulfured blackstrap molasses (optional)

A towel or mat to lay on the floor, a nearby bed, or a chaise lounge chair (optional)

1. To make the coffee, use a regular, automatic drip coffeemaker just as if you were making coffee to drink. **Put 2 TBSP of organic coffee in the filter basket. Pour 1 quart plus ¼ cup of distilled or R.O. water into the coffeemaker and turn it on to make the coffee.** Do not use city tap water, as it is full of chemicals and other less-than-helpful substances. Do not use an aluminum coffee pot either, because aluminum is a toxic metal and can leach into the coffee while perking.

2. Once the coffee has been made, you should have about 1 quart of coffee, the extra ¼ cup having been absorbed into the coffee grounds. At this point, you may **add 1 TBSP of unsulfured blackstrap molasses to the entire quart while the coffee is hot and stir it in.** The molasses aids in retaining the enema and increases the efficiency of the detox effect.

3. **Let the coffee cool to body temperature.** It is acceptable to make the coffee the night before and then warm it a bit before using.

4. **Make sure the *tube* on the disposable enema bag is closed using the stopper or clamp, then open the *bag* and pour the quart of coffee into the bag.** Release the stopper or clamp and allow just enough coffee to flow into the tube so the tube is filled with coffee. If you leave the tube filled with air, you will end up pushing this air into your colon when you start the enema, and that may make it more difficult to retain the coffee.

Note: You may want to attach a rubber colon tube onto the end of the enema bag tube. A rubber colon tube is not absolutely necessary, and you can use the enema bag as is. However, some chemotherapy treatments for cancer create conditions that require up to six sets of coffee enemas a day, and since the tube on the plastic enema bag is a rather hard plastic, there is a possibility of irritating or scratching the delicate mucus membranes inside the anal opening. The rubber colon tube is much softer and gentler on these tender tissues.

If you decide to use the rubber colon tube: Look at the end of the plastic tube on the enema bag. You will see two holes... one in the *end* of the tube and a second hole on the *side* of the tube about an inch from the end. Cut off the end of the plastic tube about where the small side hole is (about 1 inch from the end). Slide the rubber colon tube onto the cut-off end of the enema bag tube, pushing the rubber as far onto it as possible, and you're ready to start.

5. **If the coffee is quite cold, run some hot water into the sink and set the bag in it for a few minutes**. This will warm it slightly to body temperature. Then hang it on your hook or shower curtain rod. In our healing rooms here at the farm, we have attached a flower-pot holder to the wall above the sink in each bathroom. The flower pot holder swings out to hold an enema bag nicely, then swings back to lie flat against the wall when not in use.

6. When preparing to begin the enema, put the towel or mat on the floor and lie on your left side with your knees drawn up, or stand at the sink, bend forward at a 45 degree angle. **Put a bit of KY jelly or oil on the end of the tube, then insert the tube slowly into the rectum about 6-9"**. If you can't get it in more than a few inches, that's okay, but be sure to let the coffee in very slowly in that case, or you may not be able to retain it.

If you are using a rubber colon tube, you should definitely use the KY jelly instead of oil. If you use oil on the rubber tube, it will not last very long. The oil will gradually affect the rubber until it is soft, sticky, loses its shape, and disintegrates. Since rubber colon tubes are relatively expensive (about $30.00) compared to the enema bag (about $5.00) taking steps to make it last is a good idea.

7. **Release the stopper or clamp and allow about 1 pint (2 cups) of coffee to slowly flow into you, then re-clamp the tube**. Pull the tube out, putting a small piece of toilet tissue around the end of the tube to catch small drips, and set it carefully in the sink or a container (bowl, can, etc.) on the sink or floor next to you, or in the tub or shower.

8. If you are already lying down, continue to **lie on your left side, holding the coffee in the rectum for about ten minutes before expelling**. At first it may be difficult to retain the enema, but with experience you will be able to hold it with considerable ease.

If you insert the coffee while standing up at the sink, find a place to rest, relax, and if possible, lie on your side after the coffee is in. This could be either on the floor, a nearby bed, or a chaise lounge chair. Here at home, I have a "coffee bench" built into the bathroom. The bench is 32" wide, 78" long, and is nicely padded with thick foam and a washable covering.

If you are older or physically impaired, lying on the floor may make it difficult to get up and get to the toilet in time if you should suddenly be unable to hold the coffee! Lying on a bed is an okay choice if you're sure you can hold the coffee for the entire ten minutes, but choose one that is fairly close to the toilet if you can. Sitting in a chair is also acceptable if there is no place to lie on your left side. In any case, try to lie or sit on something that allows for ease of movement when it's time to get up and go dump the coffee.

9. **After expelling the coffee into the toilet, repeat Steps 6-8, using the remaining two cups of coffee, holding for ten minutes, then expelling.**

10. When you are finished with the second pint of coffee, **rinse out the bag, washing the end of the colon tube with warm, soapy water. Hang the bag to dry** on a clothes hanger or hook in open air in an inconspicuous place.

11. **Wash your bottom, and wipe off the underside of the toilet seat, and you are finished.**

If you have had a colostomy, you can still do a coffee enema as part of a detox routine to keep your liver functioning. When doing a coffee enema with a colostomy, it is necessary to lie down on your side instead of stand. Then, insert the tube from the enema bag into the colostomy opening about 6 inches, and *very slowly* release about 1 cup of coffee into the colon. Some people have worked their way up to two cups, but even one cup will do the job. My experience with colostomies is that people who have them very quickly train their colon to empty at the same time every day in order to make clean-up easier. Thus, you can train yourself to hold onto a coffee for ten minutes. During these ten minutes, replace the colostomy bag, and then release the coffee into the colostomy bag. Your liver will respond just as well as if you were introducing coffee into the rectum. Empty the colostomy bag, rinse it, and reuse it for the second coffee enema in the set. It's a little more work than doing a coffee without a colostomy, but the health benefits are well worth it.

❖

When doing coffee enemas, a few people who have never been coffee drinkers may feel slightly jittery at first, although most people quickly find the enemas very relaxing. Usually, the jitteriness lessens after about the third session. If the jitteriness continues, try adding the molasses to it, which adds minerals, aids retention, and usually leaves you calm. If you are still jittery afterwards, you are making the coffee too strong. Visually the coffee should look like light brown water and works very well at this strength.

I have read a variety of instructions for making the coffee to be used in a coffee enema and was quite surprised to find that some instructions said to put one quart of water in a pan with a cup of ground coffee and let it boil!! My personal opinion is that this is much too strong. The body is not a stupid or unresponsive organism. It will respond in just minutes to the *energy* of even homeopathic-strength coffee introduced rectally.

The reason for doing a coffee enema in the first place is that there is a sympathetic resonance between the liver and the colon. Putting weak coffee into the rectum induces the liver to dump its wastes into the colon, which then expels them into the toilet. "Doing a coffee," as I refer to it, has a powerful effect on the liver. If you do not remember anything else about coffee enemas, remember this: *you do not do a coffee to clean out your colon. You do a coffee because it detoxifies the liver.* When the coffee enters the rectal opening, it immediately causes the liver to start a series of gentle contractions that dump toxins and metabolic waste, gradually promoting better liver function.

As mentioned in an earlier chapter, people who have cancer and are getting chemotherapy can get very sick. If this is true for you, you may do up to 12 coffee enemas a day while the body is breaking down and disposing of dead cancer tissue. That's six sets, or 1 set every four hours, which seems like a lot until you consider that it serves to keep the liver from being overwhelmed and shutting down. If the liver shuts down, death is imminent.

The coffee enema is one of your most useful tools for healing! I recommend doing a coffee enema any time there is flu, fever, PMS or premenstrual headaches, nausea, many kinds of illness, during the early stages of a new exercise program, or any kind of difficulty that leaves you feeling full of aches, pains, and fatigue.

During a full detox program in which there is not a life-threatening situation, the usual recommendation is to do at least one set of coffee enemas every single day for the full length of the repair and rebuild program. The coffees can be done in the morning, the late afternoon, or early evening. This can last up to five years if you have committed to complete reversal of a serious condition.

Once you are past a crisis or have completed your rebuilding and enter into everyday maintenance of your health, various options are available. You might do coffees for one week out of every month, or perhaps only when you are doing one of the major detox routines such as a Liver Flush or Colon Sweep. You might do them two or three times a week. You might do them every other week. The idea is to do them enough to keep the liver at a peak of function, or at least to provide relief when it is overwhelmed with the waste material of illness.

One of the fears you may hear about doing enemas over a long period of time is that you will become dependent on them and won't be able to have a bowel movement without an enema. While this may be true for laxatives, I have found that it is not true with coffee enemas. The diet of whole foods that are required for you to heal contains large amounts of fiber, and this guarantees that your bowels will continue to work without problems. Even after very long periods of coffee enemas, the most sluggish of bowels takes only a day or two to work on its own. For many people on a real food diet with its high amounts of fiber, it is not uncommon to have a bowel movement on their own on days when they also do a coffee enema. Each of us is different, and thus each will use the coffee enema a little differently. Regardless of how and when it is used, the great value of a coffee enema is its ability to detox and clear the liver, which boosts its filtering action and keeps you healthy and energized. ❖

21
Chelation

I AM NOT AN EXPERT on chelation therapies, but I have had to learn the basics about them for my own healing and will pass this on to you because the truth surrounding this technique is very important.

There are two kinds of chelation therapy: EDTA and DMPS.

EDTA (ethylene-diamine-tetra-acetic acid) chelation is an intra-venous procedure used to remove plaque and sclerotic material from arteries and veins, thus improving circulation and eliminating the need for heart bypass surgery, reducing the risk of heart attacks and strokes, and improving oxygen to the brain which, in turn, improves memory, brain function, and clarity of thinking.

Chelation also helps to speed healing over a very broad spectrum because improved circulation improves delivery of nutrients to all areas of the body and delivers oxygen to all parts of your system. Oxygen is the most potent antibiotic known to man and promotes healing of all tissues.

This form of chelation is done at a clinic where a patient or client sits in a chair while the EDTA chemical is introduced into the body intravenously for about an hour. The therapy works best if the patient goes for treatment about three times a week for roughly ten to twelve weeks every two years. A good, high nutrition diet, regular exercise, avoidance of sugar – which makes the blood sticky and more prone to heart attack – and the practice of routine detox, especially the liver flush, should accompany chelation. When it does, veins and arteries are cleared, the risk of heart attack or stroke is greatly reduced, and the body begins to rebuild a strong, healthy circulatory system.

There has been a great deal of misinformation about EDTA chelation, and stories of quackery have attempted to discredit this important healing technique. Some say the medical profession is attempting to protect the high incomes made by doctors who are in the business of bypass surgery. While this may hold some truth, it is just as likely that most doctors are acutely aware of the dangers of heart attack and do not want to take the risk that someone may have a serious heart attack while they are responsible for that individual.

Of course, when there's an emergency and a heart attack is in progress, chelation is not appropriate and the techniques and surgeries that characterize "rescue medicine" are invaluable. Also, since doctors have it drilled into them again and again that they are responsible for their patient's lives – and they pay exorbitant malpractice fees to protect themselves while taking on this responsibility – they don't like to utilize therapies that don't provide the instant fix that relieves their own worries about a patient's condition. Remember, when you visit an MD, he becomes responsible for your health – not you.

In addition, since many doctors know almost nothing about nutrition and detox, they don't understand chelation, and therefore can't use it effectively. Neither can they use the fasting, foods, and supplements that create such powerful effects in the human body/mind system. This is changing, albeit slowly, and in the future, I suspect more and more doctors who are interested in real healing will include chelation, detox, and high nutrition, will come to trust these in helping to heal the human body/mind system.

DMPS (dimercapto propanesulfonic acid) chelation is used when it is necessary to remove heavy metals and toxic chemicals from the body quickly. Over the last 50 years, we have been poisoning our world and ourselves in thousands of ways, with heavy metals such as cadmium, mercury, lead, arsenic, aluminum, nickel, cobalt, and many others. Over 63,000 different chemicals such as DES, various nitrates and nitrites, aspartame, aflatoxins, MSG, antibiotics, BHA, PCBs, chlorine, cyclamates, DDT, diazinon, dozens of preservatives, and a host of "natural" flavorings are accumulating in our bodies where they derange hormones, cause serious degenerative diseases, and interfere with our blood's capacity to carry many nutrients and oxygen. [66] [67]

Let's take mercury, since it is quite common in our mouths in the form of mercury-silver amalgams (50% mercury/30% silver) used to fill cavities in teeth. [68] Research has shown that mercury oxidizes from the average person's amalgam fillings at the rate of 150 mcg. per day! [69] When dentists order, store, and dispose of the mercury-silver compound they use to fill teeth, they must follow strict federal guidelines for the handling of hazardous, toxic materials. [70] Yet, once it's in someone's mouth, the claim of the American Dental Association is that it's harmless.

Unfortunately, this is not true. When molecules of mercury oxidize and break away from the filling, they are breathed into the lungs, absorbed into mucus membranes in the mouth, or combined with food and swallowed into the gastrointestinal system. From these points of entry, the mercury gets into the brain, the blood, and even crosses the placenta in a pregnant woman and can do its damage within minutes. [71]

Once in the blood, molecules of mercury either sit on the docking sites that would normally hold oxygen, or the mercury causes hemoglobin molecules to swell and twist out of shape. Once twisted, oxygen cannot dock on the molecule of hemoglobin. Since a shortage of oxygen immediately creates a shortage of energy, you will suffer from fatigue. Since oxygen is also a powerful antibiotic, you are more susceptible to colds, flu, and other diseases going around your community. [72]

Heavy metals that get into your gastrointestinal system wreak havoc there as well. Staphylococcus and streptococcus organisms live naturally in your gut because their job is to break down the remains of the food you eat and prepare it to be eliminated. When a staph or strep molecule meets a heavy metal, it is immediately aware that its existence is under threat from the frequencies and effects of the heavy metal. So it

---

[66] Paavo Airola PhD, *How To Get Well* (Sherwood, OR: Health Plus Publishers, 1993) p. 167-177.
[67] *Acres USA News,* Acres USA Publishing.
[68] Hal Huggins DDS, MA, *It's All in Your Head* (Garden City Park, NY: Avery Publishing Group, 1993) p. 23-24
[69] Huggins, p. 35.
[70] Huggins, p. 36-37
[71] Huggins, p. 33.
[72] Huggins, p. 105-106.

runs to a neighboring cell, steals or "borrows" the DNA from that cell, and then has enough DNA to out-maneuver any antibiotic by mutating with astonishing rapidity. The result is an infectious "super bug" that can resist anything we can throw at it. [73] When you consider that staph and strep bacteria also live in the soil, where we spray all kinds of toxic pesticides, herbicides, and fungicides all stabilized with heavy metals, you can see why the super bugs have become a real threat in our world.

In my opinion, this is why we have so many antibiotic-resistant drugs. There may be some truth to the idea that too many antibiotics are being given and this is how bacteria become resistant, but this is mostly conjecture. The real culprit is the use of heavy metals in pesticides, herbicides, fungicides, and the thousands of other chemicals in our world today, which we then ingest and suffer the effects of.

If you are not healing properly after doing all the right things, including exercise, good nutrition, the right supplements and herbs, and a good detox routine, you may need chelation therapy to remove heavy metals. You cannot heal if you have too many heavy metals in you because they so powerfully distort the repair efforts of the body. There are good clinics around the country. Ask around. You can find a good one. ❖

---

[73] Huggins, p. 55.

Part 4

Supplements

22

Enzymes and Glandulars

ONCE UPON A TIME, not so very long ago, a young man named Ed Howell graduated from college and went out in the world to work. He didn't get very far with his career, however, because he was so tired, so fatigued, and so sick that he couldn't get himself out of bed in the morning. He did everything he knew to heal himself and get going with his life, but nothing worked. He went to one doctor after another, but no one was able to help him. As a last resort, he checked into a place he had heard of in Illinois, a place where only "health nuts" and the desperate went. It was a place where the emphasis was on diets using raw foods and other nutritional therapies.

To his surprise, he began to feel better. When he asked the head of the institution what secret they were using to create such miraculous results, the doctor said, "Enzymes." It was the direction Ed Howell was to pursue for the rest of his life.[74] He obtained a degree in medicine, joined the staff of the Lindlahr Sanitarium, and later started the Food Enzyme Research Foundation. Over his life, he designed and carried out a number of powerful research projects which showed conclusively that pancreatic enzymes were largely responsible for continuously rebuilding

---

[74] Dr. Nicholas Gonzales MD, from a lecture given at Boulder Colorado Medical Center, Boulder, CO, March, 1992.

and repairing the body, and that many, if not all, degenerative diseases that humans suffer and die from are caused by the body's slowing production of pancreatic enzymes.

Every living thing, be it a plant, an animal, or a human, is alive because of enzymes. *Enzymes are life energy,* and scientists have been unable to synthesize them. Without enzymes you would die quickly.

"Enzymes are the substances that make life possible. They are needed for every chemical reaction that takes place in the human body. No mineral, vitamin, or hormone can do any work without enzymes. Our bodies, all of our organs, tissues, and cells, are run by metabolic enzymes. They are the manual workers that build our body from proteins, carbohydrates, and fats, just as construction workers build our homes. You may have all the raw materials with which to build, but without the workers (enzymes) you cannot even begin." [75]

Says Stephan Blauer, "Without the life energy of enzymes, we would be nothing more than a pile of lifeless chemical substances— vitamins, minerals, water, and proteins." [76]

Everything we do...working, sleeping, breathing, healing, and more, depends on our ability to produce enzymes, and in this effort the pancreas is the key producer. "Indeed, each of us could be regarded as an orderly, integrated succession of enzyme reactions." [77]

In his small but spectacular book, *Enzyme Nutrition,* Howell wrote:

> "The living body is under a great daily burden to produce the volume of enzymes necessary to run efficiently... (and) enzymes are continually being used and eliminated in the urine, feces, and sweat. The laboratory in every hospital can find them there. They are needed in digesting food; running the heart, kidneys, liver, and lungs; and even in thinking.
>
> "Life could not exist without enzymes. Enzymes convert the food we eat into chemical structures that can

---

[75] Edward Howell, *Enzyme Nutrition* (Wayne, NJ: Avery Publishing Group, 1985) p. 33.
[76] Howell, p. ix.
[77] Howell, p. 33.

pass through the cell membranes of the cells lining the digestive tract and into the bloodstream." [78]

❖

There are basically three kinds of enzymes...

1. Metabolic Enzymes are used to rebuild and repair the human body, as well as run many of the ongoing reactions that take place within us. At present, science estimates that there are at least 6,000 metabolic enzyme systems in the body, and perhaps as many as 10,000. I call these enzymes "R&R" enzymes because they are essential for the constant *repair and rebuilding* that goes on.

2. Digestive Enzymes are those produced by the body specifically to help digest food that we eat. I separate digestive enzymes into two broad categories: stomach enzymes and intestinal enzymes. The most widely known digestive enzymes are protease, amylase, lipase, and cellulase. Protease is used to digest protein, amylase digests carbohydrates, lipase is for digesting fats, and cellulase digests cellulose, part of the structure of green plants.

3. Food Enzymes are enzymes that exist naturally in whole foods before they are cooked, baked, fried, or otherwise processed. All fresh foods contain complete sets of highly specialized enzymes designed to help the body digest that food so its nutrients and nutritional co-factors will be made available to the body. These enzymes are provided by nature to assist in the digestion of that food so the body does not have to spend its precious life energy producing digestive enzymes and can be free to concentrate on the continuous work of repair and rebuilding. For instance, raw milk has the enzymes lactase, catalase, galactase, amylase, oleinase, peroxidase, dehydrogenase, and phospha-tase, among others, all designed to help you digest the milk once you drink it. [79]

Enzymes are very sensitive to heat and begin to die when the temperature of the food goes above 117° F. [80] You can hold your hand in water at temperatures below 117° F, but when the water goes above that,

---

[78] Howell, p. 33.
[79] Howell, p. 36.
[80] Howell, p. 72.

it begins to sting and become quite uncomfortable. This is a convenient test for whether or not something is hot enough to destroy enzymes. [81]

The enzymes in fruits, vegetables, grains, and meats don't stand a chance in our highly industrialized food processing industries. And as if that weren't enough, cooking and baking temperatures in the modern kitchen are very high, and the result is complete destruction of the enzymes in anything that is cooked. Most food enzymes are destroyed by the time the food reaches 140° F, and the destruction of any remaining life energy is complete by 180° F.

When we eat cooked foods, there are no living enzymes left in it to help the digestion process. From this, it should be clear that if your pancreas has to stop producing R&R enzymes in order to start producing digestive enzymes, then the body has to suspend or at least cut back its repair and rebuilding processes. In short, the body's continuous healing program slows drastically, and may even come to a halt whenever we eat cooked or processed food.

If eating were a temporary and occasional interruption, we might overlook it. But think about what happens for millions of us every day. It takes anywhere from one to six hours to digest cooked or processed food. During this time, the body's effort to repair and rebuild itself is seriously compromised, if not halted. If you are one of the many people who snack endlessly throughout the day, sometimes right up to the time you go to bed at night, your body will be too busy trying to deal with what you are putting in your mouth to focus on the structures and processes it needs to repair. You then have the foundation for a slow-but-sure degeneration of the body, just like an old house that no one bothers to take care of any more.

If you are interested in serious healing, adding digestive enzymes to your daily diet is very important. Doing so helps the healing process immeasurably by reducing the body's need to produce digestive enzymes. When it can do this, the body is free to focus on the metabolic enzymes that keep everything healthy and running smoothly.

To help your body do its best, you should know that some digestive enzymes work in the acid environment of the stomach, and others work in the alkaline environment of the intestine, and you will probably need both. Of course, the enzymes that come in raw food are perfectly created by nature to do an excellent job no matter what area of

---

[81] Howell, p. 5

the gastrointestinal system the food is in, but if you eat a lot of cooked food, adding enzymes to your diet is essential.

You can easily buy capsules containing protease, amylase, and lipase to take with your meals. These *digestive* enzymes tend to work in the stomach, thus they are sometimes called "stomach enzymes." Sometimes the capsule will have additional things like papain, bromelain, betaine, beet root, ox bile extract, ginger, or peppermint in it. These substances all help make the process of digestion easier and more complete so you get the full benefit of whatever nutrients are in the food without exhausting the pancreas.

You can also buy *metabolic* pancreas enzymes that do the work of both digestion and repair or rebuilding. Pancreas enzymes greatly improve your ability to absorb nutrients in the small intestine. After doing so much work to prepare the food for digestion, pancreas enzymes are a godsend in terms of their ability to help the body absorb whatever nutrition it offers.

If you have active stomach ulcers, be careful with enzymes. You may have to do a long juice fast in which you drink mainly carrot and cabbage juice in order to allow the stomach to heal before you start taking enzyme supplements. You might also avoid stomach (digestive) enzymes at first and try starting with pancreas (metabolic) enzymes for a couple of months, until your ulcers have become less troublesome and your stomach walls have repaired themselves somewhat. Chewing your food extra well will also help make up for the lack of stomach enzymes.

When you put food in your stomach, it goes into the upper area of the stomach known as the "cardiac portion" where it sits quietly for a while. During its time in the cardiac area, the food enzymes in the food (if any) continue the all-important process of pre-digestion, which actually begins in the mouth when you chew the food and douse it with saliva. Fruits stay in the cardiac portion for 15 to 20 minutes if they are raw, longer if canned or cooked. Vegetables like peas, broccoli, lettuces, and tomatoes stay in the stomach for up to an hour if raw, up to two hours if cooked. Carbohydrates like bread, cereal, and pasta stay in the stomach for two to three hours, while meats, cheeses, other dairy products, and nuts stay in the stomach for three to six hours.

As the enzymes in the food – plus any stomach enzymes you've taken – successfully predigest the chewed food, known at this point as "chyme," some of the food begins to sink into the lower portion of the stomach where it soaks in the stomach acid known as hydrochloric acid

(HCL) and where the peristaltic churning of the lower stomach continues to prepare the food for the remaining journey through the gastro-intestinal system.

The importance of enzymes cannot be overstated. If everything you eat comes out of a box, bag, can, or jar, you are, in effect, levying a heavy enzyme tax on your body because the body must produce extra enzymes to make up for what is missing in the food. [82] You might consider this to be a 50% tax since the effect on the body is to shorten life by half. Since the body is designed to easily last ten times your age at puberty, most of us should be living to at least 120 years of age.

Obviously this is not the case. Many of us are dead and buried by the age of 75. This is why our governments and institutions have no wisdom and no long-term perspective in them. We die too early and never live to see the long-term effects of our decisions, processes, and creations. We are gone before we have a chance to learn anything.

I see lives in terms of "thirds." We spend the first third of our lives gathering information and learning how this reality we were born into works.

Around age 40, we move into the second third of life, and just as we should be reaping some of the benefits of our long tutelage… just as we enter our power and should begin applying what we have learned… we start falling apart with fatigue, high blood pressure, diabetes, cancers, heart disease, arthritis, and other physical nightmares.

Of course, the third "third," which begins around the age of 70, doesn't have a chance! We are gone without ever having time to evaluate or assess whether what we created is working without disastrous long-term effects. Time for reflection is gone. We settle for short-term effects because the term of our life is so short. Too often, we look at something that has been working for a relatively short time and decide it is good. We then assume it will work forever. It is always convenient to make a decision once and not have to pay attention to it after that, but this is a poor strategy for surviving and thriving. If all our attention is caught up in coping with a body that is falling apart, we have no time or energy for changes within the larger system that require more time and energy.

❖

---

[82] Howell, p. 81.

Your body has an endocrine system of strategically placed glands whose job it is to manufacture the various chemicals that will then trigger specific activities and reactions in the body. The main glands in this system are the pituitary, hypothalamus, thyroid, parathyroids, thymus, pancreas, liver, adrenals, ovaries, and testicles. The pituitary is the master gland that often sends commands to the other glands in the endocrine system.

The pituitary and hypothalamus are closely connected to the operations of the brain and are responsible for managing some of the most basic balance points, such as the body's need for oxygen and water, our fight-or-flight response, and many emotional and perceptual states.

The thyroid is heavily involved in digestion and absorption processes, as well as helping maintain steady energy and body temperature, and a host of general body operations from the sex drive to attitude.

The parathyroid glands are responsible for the metabolism of calcium in the body, which affects all muscle movement, including the heart muscle.

The thymus is the main player in the immune system and its many functions, whereas the pancreas is the main center for production of thousands of enzymes and their work in the body.

The adrenals not only regulate many heart activities, they produce the chemicals that allow us to cope with stress. And the ovaries and testicles are key players in our ability to reproduce.

In addition to the glandular substances produced by the endocrine system, your organs also create chemical instructions for each other and for all of the systems of the body, especially the brain, heart, kidneys, liver, spleen, lungs, and reproductive organs. These chemical messengers not only carry out the functions of the body, they also help create the emotional states and feelings that accompany or trigger the actions themselves.

For instance, when estrogen levels are high, a woman will feel much more romantically inclined. When thyroxin levels are high, she will have enough energy to go to work all day and clean closets all night, even if her family complains that she is disturbing them.

Sometimes aging will slow the activity of glands, and sometimes a disease process interferes with their work, but in today's world of toxic materials, oxygen-deprived air, poisoned water, dead soil, and foods empty of any nutrition, the most common causes of poor glandular activity are interference from heavy metals and an absence of nutritional factors that would allow ongoing repair and rebuilding of the glands. Once your glands begin to falter, the production of hormones, neurochemicals, and enzymes that run your body begins to slip. The result is that your organs begin to malfunction. When an organ begins to malfunction, all sorts of diseases can manifest, and life can become both painful and difficult.

Taking glandulars allows the entire body to carry on with the chemical reactions that must occur to stay alive. Glandulars support both the glands themselves and the processes that the glands are responsible for inside the body. They also reduce the stress on organs by allowing many chemical sequences to continue, which keeps the body functioning while repair and rebuilding goes on. The effect is to reduce or eliminate the tendency for diseases to become an entire string of difficulties, each one triggering the next in a sequence of breakdowns.

When designing a program to heal yourself, you often have to include several glandular supplements to support certain functions until health and balance can be re-established and the gland can take over again.

For example, if you have asthma, you would likely want to include raw lung glandulars, as well as liver and pancreas glandulars in your healing program. One lung glandular capsule each breakfast, lunch, and dinner directly supports lung function, as does the liver glandular if taken with each meal. When the liver gets sluggish or is chronically overloaded, the lungs often back up with fluids or are over-sensitive and can spasm, which leaves you coughing. Taking two to four pancreas glandular capsules with each meal supports *all* enzyme systems within the body and helps you absorb nutrients from your food, thus these three glandulars would prove to be very powerful assistants toward healing.

In another example, if you have heart trouble, you may want to add raw heart glandular, along with liver, adrenal, and pancreas glandulars. The liver and pancreas would be taken for the same reasons given above, whereas the heart and adrenal glandulars would support normal heart function.

If you have cysts on your ovary, a healing program might include raw ovary, pancreas, and liver glandulars.

If you have osteoporosis, you might want to include pituitary, pancreas, and liver glandulars on your supplement list. If the osteoporosis is severe, you might want to get injections of Human Growth Hormone (HGH), a powerful glandular that increases bone density and muscle mass, while greatly improving lung function and health in general. [83] Since bone density will also increase greatly in response to exercise, the HGH glandular plus a regular exercise program will do wonders for the problem of bones that break any time sudden pressure is applied to them.

In the case of arthritis, you might want to begin taking thyroid and parathyroid glandulars to support metabolism and the body's use of calcium, which is managed by the parathyroid glands. In addition, liver glandular supports the liver, which is a critical organ, and pancreas glandulars *greatly* reduce the pain and inflammation of arthritis.

As you may have noticed above, in almost every case of serious illness, the liver and pancreas need support, and thus these two glandular supplements are frequently included in a good healing program. This is especially true of cancers, since the *pancreatic enzymes trypsin and chymotrypsin will directly dissolve the fibrin covering that shields tumors and cancers from the immune system,* thus allowing your own killer cells to get at the cancerous growth and destroy it.

Dr. William Kelley's healing program suggests that people with cancer get up at 2:30 am to take nearly a dozen pancreas glandular capsules because the pancreas itself is very active at that time of the day. The combined effect of what the pancreas puts out, plus the dozen pancreas capsules, overwhelms cancers and tumors, killing them outright and breaking them down. The liver then filters the dead tumor tissue out of the blood so it can be excreted. Generally speaking, in cases of cancer, you might take an entire complex of glandulars plus extra amounts of thymus and spleen glandulars in order to break down tumors, support the immune system, assist the body's ability to make new blood, and to repair itself perfectly. [84]

It is highly recommended that you do not take pancreas glandulars and enzymes to dissolve a cancer unless you also embark on a full detox program. I would like to emphasize again that dead, dissolving tumor tissue is *extremely* poisonous and will quickly overwhelm the liver. If the liver gets plugged, you will be very ill. If it shuts down and you don't get it functioning again, you can die quickly. Constantly

---

[83] James F. Balch MD and Phyllis A. Balch CNC, *Prescriptions for Natural Healing* (Garden City Park, NY: Avery Publishing Group, 1997) p. 552-553.
[84] Teaching of Dr. Nicholas Gonzales MD.

detoxifying the liver and lymph system becomes a steady challenge and requires daily coffee enemas plus a continuous rotation through the major detox routines of Liver Flush, Colon Sweep, and Purge on a monthly, or even bi-weekly, basis until the cancer is gone.

We have all heard of people who started a chemotherapy program for cancer and then died from the effects of the chemo. Now you know why! The chemo kills the cancer, along with a lot of other living tissue in the body. Both the dead cancer tissue and the chemicals used in chemotherapy are highly poisonous substances in themselves. The liver is seldom given the support it needs to handle the onslaught of dead and toxic material that accumulates in the body during chemotherapy treatments. The result is that the entire body/mind system weakens terribly and sometimes gives up. Much of this can be avoided with the practice of detox and a good supplement program consisting of enzymes, glandulars, amino acids, minerals, and vitamins. Together, these constitute a key part in getting well again naturally. So, let's do a quick review of what the amino acids, minerals, and vitamins actually do. ❖

23
Amino Acids, Minerals, and Vitamins

IT HAS BEEN KNOWN for a very long time that any group of people who wish to survive must eat a combination of foods that will supply all of the amino acids that the body uses to create the entire array of proteins needed for the body to survive. There are usually key foods in any given culture that become staples simply because they provide the essential amino acids that are not found elsewhere.[85] For Japanese, it is rice and fish. For Mexicans, it is beans and corn. For Americans, it is meat, milk, and potatoes.

If you want your body to be able to produce enzymes and gland, you have to get enough amino acids in your diet. In fact, in the hierarchy of supplements, amino acids are at the top of the list.

Amino acids are needed to utilize...

Minerals, which are needed to utilize...

Vitamins, all of which are needed to produce...

Enzymes, which run the body and are necessary for making...

---

[85] The key word here is *essential*, which means the body cannot make these amino acids for itself and they must be supplied from the diet. Since not every food contains these essential amino acids, certain foods become critical because they supply the missing aminos, without which, civilization would die out.

Glandulars (aka hormones), the major players in your endocrine system that act as chemical on-off switches!

In fact, all of these elements are intimately interconnected. You can't utilize minerals without the correct amino acids, and you can't use vitamins well without all the necessary minerals. The bottom line is that you will have great difficulty producing certain enzymes and glandulars without the proper amino acids, minerals, and vitamins, and you need *enough* of each in the entire bunch to run the body properly and maintain physical, mental, emotional, and spiritual health.

Amino acids are the critical building blocks used to make a human body. Aminos are the pieces and parts used to create proteins in their thousands of forms. For instance, hair and toenails are protein, muscles are protein, your glands are made of protein, your blood is protein, and so are many of the tissues, fluids, and organs that make up your body.

When you eat food with proteins in it, your body breaks down the proteins that once formed the body of the plant or animal you are eating, turning it into its original molecular form of vitamin, mineral, and amino acid components. It then recycles these components to build its own highly specialized proteins, each of which has unique uses and applications.

Amino acids can run short in your body if you are under stress, are suffering from a trauma or infection of any kind, are getting older, have impaired absorption of nutrients, take drugs – including over-the-counter and prescription drugs, or have a poor diet characterized by too much sugar, too little fiber, and too few nutrients.

The body can produce about 80% of the amino acids it needs, but the rest must come from your diet. Without the needed types or sufficient amounts of amino acids, you can easily fall prey to illness and disease. If you don't pay attention to the warnings of nutrient deficiency, you are liable to develop an entire cascade of problems, each one feeding on the one before it, complicating the situation immensely.

When you buy amino acids, look for the words *free-form amino acids* on the label, which means that the aminos do not have to be digested or worked on by the body and are ready for absorption directly into your bloodstream. You can also look for a statement that says the aminos came from organic sources and are *L-form* aminos, which has a left-hand molecular spin, (as opposed to D-form, which have a right-hand spin) so that they are more useable by your body. And make sure that the full set of aminos is included in the capsule or powder you buy. There are nine essential aminos, which your body cannot make and must get from food or supplements.

These nine essential aminos are:

Histidine improves digestion, increases interest in sexual activity, is used in growth and repair of tissues, helps remove heavy metals and protect from radiation.

Methionine helps prevent fat build-up in arteries and the liver, is a potent antioxidant and detox agent, helps excrete excess estrogen, is important in cell building and maintaining muscle strength, assists in reducing allergic reactions and preventing osteoporosis, and increases the energy of cell metabolism.

Isoleucine maintains energy and endurance, is used in making new tissues including hemoglobin, and stabilizes blood sugar.

Leucine promotes healing of bones, skin, and tissues; is used to produce Growth Hormone; and provides energy for the body's use.

Phenylalanine is used by the body to synthesize neurotransmitters, which are utilized by the brain; helps with alertness, memory, and learning; keeps appetite down and spirits up; helps with everything from PMS to Parkinson's disease; and even works to control pain.

Lysine is used to improve and manage calcium absorption; fights cold sores and herpes outbreaks; assists the immune system in building antibodies; aids tissue repair, collagen formation, and muscle formation; lowers triglycerides; helps the body build enzymes; prevents hair loss and irritability; keeps energy up; maintains reproductive ability; and prevents anemia.

Threonine assists liver function, prevents fatty deposits, keeps proteins in balance, forms collagen, and is used in a number of key organs like the heart and brain.

Tryptophan is used by the body to synthesize serotonin, stabilize moods, relieve migraines, reduce appetite, fight insomnia and depression, reduce stress, manage hyperactivity in children, and maintain correct coronary artery tension.

Valine is used as an energy source, maintains nitrogen balance in the body thus improving cell construction, and helps with tissue repair.

The remaining amino acids:

Alanine is used to metabolize glucose in the body.

Arginine is important for tumor control, muscle metabolism, and production of pancreatic enzymes; builds bones, tissue, muscle, and collagen; triggers sexual maturity; enhances immune function; and helps produce a variety of hormones and enzymes.

Asparagine helps create balance in the nervous system and in transforming other amino acids into useful forms.

Aspartic acid enhances immune function, removes toxins from the blood, assists DNA and RNA functions, prevents disorder in the brain and central nervous system, and reduces fatigue.

Citrulline is a detoxifying agent and helps release energy in the body. It supports arginine's efforts to retard tumors and cancers, and is an overall stimulant to the immune system.

Cysteine & Cystine are two closely related and very important aminos in terms of their detox effects. They are needed for healthy skin, hair, eyes, collagen, and digestive enzymes; help fight cancers and arthritis; promote healing; burn fats; and relieve respiratory problems.

Gamma-aminobutyric acid is known as GABA. This amino relaxes nerve activity in the body and, thus, helps with conditions like epilepsy, ADD, hypertension, anxiety, and some neuralgia.

Glutamic acid is used as a neurotransmitter and is important in the metabolism of carbohydrates and fats. It also transports potassium, can serve as fuel for the brain, and improves nerve action and reaction.

Glutamine is a key amino needed for brain function and good mental activity; helps detoxify the brain; builds good muscle and connective tissue; is essential for maintaining DNA, the digestive tract, and acid/alkaline balance in the body. Glutamine reduces cravings for sugar, and is useful for treating everything from alcoholism and arthritis to ulcers, MS, impotence, and senility.

Glycine helps the body synthesize other amino acids; builds muscle tissue; maintains DNA and RNA; and promotes conditions like a healthy prostate, good digestion, and fast repair of injured tissues.

Ornithine promotes production of growth hormone, aids in detoxification of the liver, and supports the synthesis of other amino acids in the body.

Proline helps create a strong heart, good connective tissues and tendons, healthy joint capsules, and good skin.

Serine is used in the body's metabolism of fats and as a major support for the immune system.

Taurine, another key amino in the body, promotes utilization of the six major minerals: calcium, magnesium, sodium, potassium, zinc, and iron, as well as trace minerals. It helps produce bile, which allows digestion of fats, which in turn allow absorption of fat-soluble vitamins. This amino also supports everything from a steady, even heartbeat, good eyesight, and healthy cholesterol levels to healthy blood, muscles, and brain function.

Tyrosine aids in raising your mood and keeping depression at bay while suppressing your appetite and burning fat. It assists the thyroid, reduces fatigue, eases chronic headaches, Parkinson's disease, and allergies.

For a more complete discussion of amino acids, read the section on Amino Acids in *Prescription For Nutritional Healing* by Phyllis Balch, CNC, and her husband James F. Balch, MD. This is a reference that every home should have.

Minerals – The Six Majors

In order for your body to carry on the basic processes of metabolism and the constant replenishment of basic supplies and structures, you need minerals. The basic six minerals, sometimes referred to as the *Six Majors*, that you absolutely must have on a steady basis in order to stay alive are:

Calcium is essential for good bones and teeth, keeping blood pressure down, maintaining a healthy heartbeat, lowering cholesterol, eliminating depression, and relieving literally dozens of other difficulties and conditions.

Magnesium assists the body in utilizing calcium and potassium. It's also needed for a smoothly working nervous system; to provide support for enzyme systems; and help prevent osteoporosis, PMS, and depression as well as many other irritating conditions.

Sodium supports the work of the stomach, nerves, and muscles; maintains proper blood pressure; keeps the liver and kidneys healthy while helping to prevent a wide variety of symptoms such as depression, confusion, poor memory, gas, headache, loss of coordination, infections, and lack of energy.

Potassium is a co-worker of sodium that aids nerve and muscle function, especially the heart. It keeps blood pressure steady, helps keep the heartbeat even, maintains water balance in the body, aids respiration, keeps cells functioning normally, prevents salt retention, and assists with many of the same difficulties that sodium prevents.

Iron is necessary for high energy and a well-functioning immune system as well as for producing red blood cells and many enzymes. It helps create healthy hair, skin, and nails; prevents digestive upsets; reduces overweight and nervous irritability.

Zinc keeps the immune system healthy; promotes healing at all levels; is an ingredient in many enzyme systems; counters fatigue and lethargy; helps keep vision, taste, and smell in good working order; and is necessary to prevent infertility and impotence.

A Few Trace Minerals

Your body uses over 90 trace minerals to maintain good function. Although you can buy a good book that focuses on mineral supplements in great detail, I have listed a few here that I think are critical and well worth making sure you have in your diet.

Phosphorus is a necessary co-factor for many of the vitamins and provides a great deal of the *oompah!* in the hundreds of chemical transactions that go on in the body. It works closely with calcium and magnesium to continuously form and maintain bones and teeth. It is important for normal breathing and a steady heartbeat, for healthy, functioning kidneys and the ability to use vitamins.

Copper is necessary for your body's ability to create its cells and enzymes. It also helps keep energy and strength high, assists in all healing processes, helps maintain normal levels of triglycerides, keeps your hair from turning gray prematurely, and is necessary for zinc to do its work.

Chromium is essential in assisting your body to utilize insulin and keep blood sugar normal. It helps you metabolize amino acids, lower your cholesterol, keep weight down, and avoid osteoporosis.

Iodine is necessary to keep your thyroid gland healthy and working properly. It is needed for development and maintenance of your entire physical, mental, and emotional self. The body needs iodine in order to utilize the fats that construct both cell membranes and nerve sheathing. It also prevents fatigue and weight gain.

Manganese is a trace mineral used to build bones and keep joint capsules in good working order. It also metabolizes fats and proteins, produces important enzymes, maintains normal blood sugar, and keeps the immune system healthy.

Selenium is a powerful anti-oxidant that protects the immune system, heart, and liver; supports the pancreas; maintains fertility; and helps prevent cancer, heart disease, and liver disease.

Boron is a bone and brain enhancer that promotes the absorption of calcium thus helping you avoid osteoporosis and stay mentally sharp. It is also a co-factor in being able to keep and use other minerals within the body.

Germanium improves oxygen levels in your cells thus leading to better resistance to infection and disease. This mineral supports the immune system while acting as a detox agent in the body.

Sulfur is a basic ingredient of major amino acids and, thus, is a requirement for building every cell in your body. It is also a powerful disinfectant, acts as an anti-aging substance by keeping cell walls flexible, improves digestion and elimination, builds collagen, and protects us from radiation.

Silica works with calcium to form bones and is a key mineral in the formation of collagen and connective tissues, and in reducing arthritis and osteoporosis. It keeps you flexible and young; is necessary for healthy hair, skin, fingernails, and arteries; helps your body get rid of aluminum toxicity; and helps prevent Alzheimer's.

Molybdenum is essential for normalizing cell operations and keeping the tissues in your mouth and gums healthy. Molybdenum is important for good bones, your liver, and teeth, and helps keep male sexual potency alive and well.

Vanadium, like molybdenum, is necessary for normal cell function and for the processes that form good bones and teeth. It is also needed for reproduction, a healthy cardiovascular system, and good kidneys.

Gold is seldom thought of as a necessary mineral, but when taken as a trace element, it stabilizes mental and emotional balance while promoting a sense of well-being. It is also used as a pain-killer for burns and arthritis, to ease the difficulties of menopause, and lift the spirits of those who suffer from Seasonal Affective Disorder (SAD).

Silver is a powerful supporter of the immune system. It is effective in keeping your body clear of hundreds of viruses, fungi, and bacteria thus helping prevent and clear internal and external infections.

Vitamins

Once you have the amino acids, six major minerals, and the trace minerals in place in your diet, it is time to think about vitamins. Most people think of vitamins first and give little thought to minerals, although you must have minerals in your system before you can properly utilize vitamins.

The major oil-soluble vitamins include:

Vitamin A is known as "the healing vitamin" because without it you cannot heal, no matter what else you take or don't take. Its presence is necessary for your body to utilize protein. Since amino acids, fats, and many of the body tissues are forms of protein, Vitamin A is critical. It is essential for bone and teeth formation, protection of the major organs, good eyesight, healthy skin and mucus membranes, especially those involved in asthma, and protection from cancer.

Vitamin D is known as "the sunshine vitamin" because your body will convert cholesterol substances in your skin to Vitamin D precursors if you expose your skin to the sun for about 20 minutes three times a week. Its presence is necessary if you want to utilize the calcium you take in. It is essential for bone growth, the immune system, normal thyroid function, good eyesight, normal weight, strong muscles, and regular heartbeat.

Vitamin E is known for its protection against heart attacks and cardiovascular disease. Vitamin E not only improves your general circulation, it lowers blood pressure, promotes normal blood clotting, and repairs capillary walls. As an anti-oxidant, it preserves Vitamins A and D from attack by free radicals, preserves fertility, helps maintain vision and prevent cancers.

Vitamin K is the last of the oil-soluble vitamins (that we know of) and is required for the formation of bone and its repair. It is closely involved in the production of your body's chemical factors that maintain blood clotting ability and resistance to infections, especially ear, nose, and throat infections. It is necessary for healthy liver function, normal blood sugar, for anti-aging protection, and in preventing cancers, especially of the organs.

The major water-soluble vitamins include:

Vitamin B-Complex is a star player in the body. The B's, known as B1 (thiamin), B2 (riboflavin), B3 (niacin), B6 (pyridoxine), and B12, are involved in an extremely wide variety of functions. Usually taken together so that they are taken in the correct ratios, each is highly unique. A very partial list of their activities includes circulation, blood-building, cell building and longevity, protection of nerve sheathing, good digestion, brain function, learning capacity, good memory, good muscle tone, anti-oxidant abilities, regular heartbeat, pain reduction, good vision, healthy skin and eye tissue, normal growth rate, fertility, preventing birth defects, clear skin, stimulation of bile, production of adrenal and sex hormones, utilizing other vitamins, boosting stamina, preventing neuropathy, maintaining mental health, cancer immunity, and the production of DNA and RNA. Of them all, B-6 is a necessary ingredient in more bodily processes that any other vitamin, and without it, you will quickly go downhill.

Vitamin C is a major anti-oxidant as well as promoter of tissue repair. It also stimulates immune function and boosts iron absorption. It works as an anti-bacterial and antibiotic agent; protects against blood clotting; lowers cholesterol and blood pressure; strengthens arteries, veins, and capillary walls; and supports the immune system against infections and cancers.

Folic Acid is actually part of the B-family of water-soluble vita-mins. It is critical for being able to produce and maintain healthy blood, to prevent birth defects, in keeping the processes of protein metabolism healthy, and in helping prevent the breakdown of DNA, thus in guarding against cancer, TB, and other serious diseases.

Co-Q 10 is a powerful companion worker with Vitamin C in keeping the immune system in good working order. It helps cells to generate the energy necessary to do their work, keeps us from aging too soon, increases circulation, and is especially good for heart function.

Conditional Vitamins include:

Conditional vitamins are those that your body will manufacture under normal circumstances if deficiencies are not common. However, without the necessary amino acids, minerals, and major vitamins as building material, the body may fail to make them and problems can result.

Biotin is needed for metabolism of all major nutrients: fats and oils, carbohydrates, and proteins. It is also a key player in preventing anemia, depression, hair loss, dry or flaky skin, and pain.

Choline is another key raw ingredient in building a healthy physical body. It is used in a large number of bodily processes, especially those of the brain and nervous system, the gall bladder, and liver. It is needed for smooth, coordinated movement, for carrying fats through the blood so all cells that are in the process of rebuilding their cell membranes (which are made of a double layer of both saturated and super-unsaturated fats) will have access to these fats. Choline also helps prevent the deposit of fat in the organs of the body. It is an assistant in avoiding angina and other heart problems, ulcers, and high blood pressure.

Pantothenic Acid (B-5) is another member of the B-family. Like choline, it transports necessary fats to and from cells. It is important in the production of hormones, reducing triglycerides and cholesterol, easing stress, the development and maintenance of cartilage, and producing other important substances in the body, including antibodies, neurotransmitters, and those enzymes that manage glucose in the blood, thus assisting with prevention of diabetes.

Inositol and its total role are not yet well understood, but it is found in every single cell of the body. It is especially abundant in the heart, brain, and skeletal muscles and serves to lower cholesterol, prevent arteriosclerosis, relieve constipation, irritability, and mood swings. It also keeps fatty deposits from forming in the liver, keeps eyes healthy, helps prevent hair loss, and helps with recovery after illness.

PABA, also known as para-aminobenzoic acid, is actually a component of folic acid. Similar to the other conditional vitamins, it is essential in the metabolism of proteins. Other effects include maintaining hair color, maintaining healthy intestinal bacteria, creating normal, healthy blood cells, and preventing sunburn and skin cancer.

❖

You have now been introduced to the most basic and most familiar amino acids, minerals, and vitamins. This is not an exhaustive list by any means, it is just some of what we know so far. There are at least 75 additional trace minerals used by the body in its many and varied processes. If you eat at least some of your food as *real food* that has been grown in a healthy manner, you should be able to get many of these other trace minerals into your system.

One of the key goals of this chapter is to help you grasp the fact that your body is a self-healing system that depends on you to supply it with raw materials for repair and maintenance. These vitamins, minerals, and amino acids are another important set of tools for healing.

This is also an opportune moment to warn you against something that happens much too often. You read or hear about something that might help you with a problem you've been having, then you run out and buy that supplement and start taking it without doing your homework. Your homework is to find out what supporting supplements might be needed to make the new supplement work, and more importantly, what the cautions and contraindications might be. For instance, many of the amino acids need Vitamin B-6 to work properly.

Some people are perfect examples of the old belief that "if some is good, more is better." They buy a bottle of B-Complex capsules with 100 mg of each B-vitamin and start taking it three times a day. But be aware! Sometimes Vitamin B-6 in excess can conflict with medication taken for Parkinson's, making the medicine ineffective. This may not happen in your case, but you at least need to be aware of the possibility. All things have a *relationship* to one another! Get on the Web and do a little checking, go to the bookstore and search out a good, complete reference on vitamins and minerals, then buy it. Or go to the library and do a search there. Gradually you will learn the nature of the relationships between these substances and come to honor them.

Read, ask questions, and then experiment with the new supplement for a few weeks. If all goes well, extend the experiment for a month or two or three, *always* paying attention to what you experience and how you feel. If something comes up, read, or search for answers until you find them. If all is well, keep going, but keep your eyes open. After three weeks to three months – sometimes only three days – you should notice signs of improvement. If nothing happens after three months, your healing program needs further tweaking.

Often, vitamins do not work as well as they should because the body is so clogged with wastes. Dr. Gonzales suggests that you not even start with vitamins and minerals until you've done a complete round of detox procedures first.

Since research is ongoing and our base of information is ever-changing, this introduction to aminos, minerals and vitamins will certainly be deficient before it ever goes to press, but you have to start somewhere.

There are many other books that go more deeply into the intricacies of amino acids, minerals, and vitamin effects within the body, and if you are going to be your own healer, or be one of the healers in your family, you should have one or two of these references in your home library (see suggested references in the Appendix). Get one, read it, and work at understanding yourself as a body/mind system that functions as an integrated ecological system with many needs, checks and balances.❖

Part 5
Lifestyles and Stress

24
Foods, Moods, and Stress

IN THE EARLY DAYS, when we were still cavemen and cavewomen, our bodies developed an elaborate response to danger that was designed to help us survive. Today, our lifestyles run counter to the ways that we were designed and built to live, and this is very stressful to us. Lots of people think stress is just another vague mood, but it's not. Stress is a series of biochemical and physiological changes in the body. These changes are disastrous over time.

Imagine you are walking through the jungle and a tiger starts to chase you. This threat to your life sets in motion a chain of events called the General Adaptation Syndrome, known popularly as *stress*. The minute you recognize that you are in danger, your brain immediately downshifts from the higher brain functions found in the cortex to the mid-brain functions of the limbic system.[86] When a tiger is chasing you, you don't need to be figuring out the specific species of big cat that's chasing you or calculating the tiger's rate of approach. These are analytical activities made possible by the cortex. You *do* need to fight or run for your life, and these kinds of responses are handled in the limbic area of the brain.

---

[86] Leslie Hart, *Human Brain, Human Learning* (New Rochelle, NY: Brain Age Publishers, 1983) p.108.

Stage 1 of the stress response is alarm and begins as soon as the threat is perceived. Instantly your adrenal glands go into high gear, dumping adrenocorticotropic hormone (ACTH), cortisone, and cortisol into your bloodstream. This ACTH brings quick energy, heavy breathing, and a fast heartbeat within 30 seconds. You are immediately ready to fight or run for your life. Your blood pressure rises, and sugar pours into the bloodstream, giving quick energy to muscles and brain. Digestive processes shut down so the energy normally used to digest food can be used for defense. Red blood cells flood the arteries to take in more oxygen and dispose of carbon dioxide, while clotting factors pour into the blood to clot quickly in case the tiger bites or scratches you. Blood is withdrawn from your extremities and moved into the deep interior of the body to protect and feed vital organs and big muscle systems, and within two minutes of the start of the stress response, endorphins (brain-generated opiates) pour into the blood stream to dull perception and ease pain in case the tiger gets hold of you. The endorphins also "loosen" attention from your usual points of interest and habitual behaviors so you can move into survival mode and do whatever is required of you. The cortisone and cortisol loosen up joints and relieve stiffness, allowing you to run like a gazelle or fight with gusto.

Stage 2 of the stress response is resistance in which the fight or flight is on. During resistance, more and more of the above chemicals are released, and your body will rally intensely to defend you against the threat.

Stage 3 of the stress response is exhaustion in which your physical resources are used up, the defense and immune system wear down, and without immediate relief and attention to healing, your body gives up and dies. [87]

From this, you should be able to see that stress is not just a convenient psychological excuse for changing your life – stress is a killer. The wonderful thing about the stress response is that, if a tiger really is chasing you, it gives you the energy to run without pain (the work of the endorphins) or even a thought about being tired. If the tiger gets you (or your boss verbally blasts you), you will be so drugged by your own opiates that you may not suffer as much as usual. The bad thing about the stress response is that it is triggered whether the threat is a tiger, an angry spouse, a final exam, a rough business meeting, a screaming two-year-old, or anything else you find difficult to deal with.

---

[87] McQuade and Aikman, p. 7-9.

If you spend any amount of time in stress, not only will you exhaust your endocrine system and your immune system, you will suffer nutritionally simply because the processes of digestion shut down during stress (note *Stage 1* above). All of the nutrients you put into yourself are wasted because they are not absorbed, the body has no supplies for repair and rebuilding, the immune system is disabled, and serious degeneration sets in. This is why so many people come down with cancers, high blood pressure, diabetes, heart attacks, or other serious diseases about 1½-2 years after a period of great physical or emotional difficulty. They were caught in the stress response, and their entire body was degenerating at an extremely rapid rate. This is why you need four times the ordinary level of nutrition when you are ill or in a state of stress. The illness itself causes stress and very little nutrition is absorbed. Worse, you are using up the nutritional supplies on hand at a tremendous rate.

You should also be able to see why more heart attacks happen on Monday mornings than any other time of the week. High-pressured executives going back to work get caught in the stress response, and the clotting factors released into the blood make it easy for clots to form in veins and arteries that are already narrowed or full of plaque and other obstructions.

During periods of stress it is difficult to sleep because your endocrine system is too exhausted to produce serotonin to keep you calm or melatonin to help you sleep. Your creative abilities suffer because the downshifting of the brain from cortical to limbic functions leaves you without access to the great creative abilities of the frontal lobes of the cortex. This leaves you dull, foggy, and fatigued and interferes with your ability to see clearly what is happening around you. Thus, intelligence, decision-making, and energetic action remain just out of reach.

❖

When Weston Price was traveling the world back in the 1930s, he found that people who were getting high levels of nutrition did not experience the bad moods, petty jealousies, periods of depression, damaging competition, juvenile delinquency, or high crime that were prevalent elsewhere in society at that time and are even more so in our time. People were healthy, relaxed, creative, and cooperative. They loved the everyday processes of growing, collecting, or hunting their food. They enjoyed the personal involvement needed to gather fibers for clothing, to tan hides for pouches (purses), jackets, and other everyday items. There was no separation between art and the making of dishes, tools, blankets, rugs, or other household items needed for everyday living. A spirit of joy in their oneness with each other was expressed easily and naturally in the music, dance, and rituals that connected them to their intuition, healing abilities, wisdom of their ancestors, or the great Source that lies at the heart of everything.

Today, millions live in constant stress. Sometimes war is the cause, other times sickness or financial need is at the root of our difficulties. In many places around the globe, we are slaves to our economic system and a great deal of effort goes into making sure that system stays in place.

Many people have accepted the routine of just going to work, staying in their cubicle or rut, and repeating the one set of behaviors they were hired to do over and over and over. Yet in order to accept this kind of confinement, we must set aside, or at least seriously compromise, our need for a secure and trusting connection to Mother Nature. This compromise makes us uneasy in our soul. Worse, we are naturally creative beings, and the effort to find outlets for our creativity causes considerable stress because artificial outlets demand extra money, time, and energy. When creativity is divorced from the routines that bring us food, water, shelter, and tools, then a creative life begins to seem like a luxury instead of the necessity it really is.

The demand that we be at the office or in the factory for set, specific hours so many days in a row interferes with our freedom to travel when and where we need or want to go. The expectation that we will show up at an office or factory at the same time every day, day after day, also disrupts our natural sleep rhythms, which tend to rotate through a variety of cycles.

Sedentary lifestyles interfere with our need for full physical activity that uses the body the way it was designed to move. And all of these expectations and habits of contemporary life stress the body/mind system terribly and cause us to get old before our time. When you add the fact that the nutrition we're getting is totally inadequate, the outcome is widespread degeneration and depression that has become epidemic. We are stressed, irritable, and impatient on a regular basis.

Back in the days when we were trading tools, furs, metals, fabric, and a few specialty items directly with one another, we were somewhat on the safe side. The biggest danger was in the travel. The moment we began marketing an entire array of manufactured and artificial foods, we started down a destructive and dangerous path that is quickly leading to the collapse of our entire civilization.

No group of people has ever survived, thrived, and maintained their power on foods that do not contain the high-level nutrition required by the body. This has been the lesson for every group from the Mayans to the Romans to the Persians to the Sumerians. As I have already pointed out, get too far away from Mother Nature's soil, and you will either collapse from illness and fatigue, or someone will invade and you'll be too weak to care and too tired to defend yourself properly.

When I first started studying the mind, it led me back to the body again and again. I ignored these early observations and conclusions because I was caught up in the New Age idea that the body was just an incidental thing, completely subject to the mind. It was a long time before I realized that the mind is also subject to the body it is conjoined with. *It is a body/mind system.*

I have come to recognize that, contrary to the idea of the body as a messy, embarrassing incidental in this life, we all come here precisely to experience the great joy and sensuousness that a body offers, to create with love and enthusiasm, and to evolve that body toward full enlightenment.

Our lives are filled to the brim with the textures, tastes, sounds, feelings, sights, movements, and expressions of the body – but we are too tired and stressed to enjoy them. Yet, we are all deeply affected by what goes on around, in, and with the body. Our participation here in this reality is completely dependent on having a body to experience it with, and one of the most overlooked factors of that body is how it affects the mind.

Although most people separate physical feelings such as the pain of a stubbed toe from emotional feelings such as worry about money, the truth is that all feelings and emotions are the result of our thoughts. When we have a thought, the body then uses neurochemicals and hormones to produce feelings that match our thinking.

Although it is true that much of what you spend your life thinking about is the result of the way you've been taught to perceive and feel about reality, the fact still remains that what you feel at any given moment depends on whether or not your endocrine systems and brain can produce the chemistry that will create the feelings you would like to have, and these are the drivers that push behavior.

If your body does not have enough aminos, minerals, and vitamins with which to produce the neurochemicals that make you feel happy, sad, curious, compassionate, guilty, rushed, or any of the other emotions that are part of life, you will not be able to experience appropriate feelings or share the wholeness and richness of life. With a limited range of feelings, you end up caught in the same few emotions over and over. When this happens you become bored, angry, listless, and can behave inappropriately in situations that require a new set of feeling responses. Do this often enough as a child and you will be diagnosed as emotionally disabled, a condition that often accompanies learning disabilities. If these disabilities continue into adulthood and you fail to develop a wide enough range of sensitivity and caring, you may be labeled everything from depressed, to incompetent, to a sociopath.

You may try to develop yourself to a higher consciousness or higher levels of spirituality, but the body may not be able to respond to your intention to remain calm and loving because it does not have the supplies it needs to produce the neurochemicals that maintain a positive attitude of calm clarity, patient compassion, or loving kindness. Your moods are directly dependent on the level of nutrition you give yourself, the amount of exercise you do, and the amount of sleep you get.

If you are depressed, feel generally anxious, or have a constant sense of restlessness or irritation, it is time to survey your life and begin making changes. Although many people blame outer circumstances for their depression, if you are not superbly healthy in the first place, you will not have the energy to make needed changes in your life whether they are physical, mental, emotional, or spiritual. People who aren't healthy can't deal with the fallout resulting from inner or outer change, so they refrain from making changes at all.

To relieve stress and create or maintain a sense of emotional well-being and balance, all of the things we have talked about in this book are critically important. This includes changing your diet to real foods, detoxing your body regularly, balancing your amino acid, vitamin, and mineral intake, avoiding foods that you are allergic to, making sure you are *absorbing* the nutrition you're taking in, and getting enough general exercise as well as aerobic exercise.

Be sure you are getting enough of the right fats – saturated and superunsaturated – because you need these to utilize the major, oil-soluble vitamins. Avoid eating a low-fat diet because this quickly causes depression, irritability, unsocial behavior, fatigue, and a host of conditions characterized by mental or emotional degeneration.

If you live a highly stressed life, you may be deficient in amino acids, magnesium, calcium, Vitamin B-6, and the entire Vitamin B-Complex, as well as the essential fats Omega 3 and 6.

It is important to avoid all white sugar/white flour products, and at least one meal a day should consist of raw foods. Either eat fruit all morning or a very large salad with lots of vegetables in it for lunch or dinner. Extra tyrosine, glutamine, tryptophan, or phenylalanine, or methionine may also be needed, depending on the specific and individual symptoms of the depression.

Sometimes the depression is mild and we just feel stressed and irritable all the time. In his book, *Nutrition and The Mind*, Gary Null quotes Dr. Lendon Smith as saying…

> "What we've found is that if their level of GGT (a liver and gallbladder enzyme called gamma glutamil transpeptidase) is below 20, they're more likely to have some of these magnesium deficiency symptoms—short attention span, trouble relaxing or sleeping, little muscle cramps in the feet and legs, a craving for chocolate. Most of these people don't like to be touched. They may be a little crabby. (All of these) symptoms go with low magnesium… which is one of the first minerals to disappear from food when it's been processed. Magnesium is also one of the first minerals to leave the body when there is stress, which accounts for how so many women behave a day or two before their periods. They feel stressed because they're losing their magnesium."[88]

Good nutrition is a non-negotiable factor in your life as well as a miracle worker. Even the more challenging mental problems such as bipolar disorder, schizophrenia, alcoholism, ADHD, autism, chronic fatigue syndrome, pre-menstrual syndrome, aggressive behavior, Alzheimer's, anorexia, and bulimia respond well and sometimes disappear with high-density nutrition, a good diet, and exercise.

If you are constantly fatigued more than depressed, you're probably deficient in light exercise, amino acids, magnesium, calcium, the entire Vitamin B-Complex, iron, and potassium. You may need DMPS chelation and might also benefit from any therapy that increases oxygen, such as ½ TSP of hydrogen peroxide in a cup of water every

---

[88] Null, p. 42.

day, or a gingko biloba supplement, which improves circulation and increases delivery of nutrients to the tissues. One caution – do not take iron and hydrogen peroxide together as they cancel and complicate one another. I would take the iron first for about a month, then switch to hydrogen peroxide for a month, then back to iron for another month, then to hydrogen peroxide again, moving back and forth between the two. It helps build reserves of energy without the complications. And sometimes, the iron does the entire task.

Manic depression, known today as bipolar disorder, is often the result of the body's inability to metabolize zinc properly. Often, there is a need for the natural mineral lithium, extra Vitamin B-Complex, the right combination of fats, and the complete set of amino acids.

Schizophrenia responds slowly but well to a full detox program, complete elimination of sugar, elimination of all foods that the body is allergic to, Vitamin B-12, Vitamin B-3, Vitamin C, the entire Vitamin B-Complex, calcium, magnesium, zinc, manganese, chromium, selenium, amino acids, acidophilus, pancreas enzymes, raw butterfat (from milk or butter), Omega 3 and 6 fats, drinking distilled water regularly, and ½-1 TSP of ordinary 3% hydrogen peroxide in a glass of water, plus regular exercise. [89]

It would also help if the extraordinary abilities that schizophrenic people have for dipping into other dimensions of reality could be shaped, channeled, or put to good use rather than dismissing this skill as craziness. Schizophrenia is a problem in bio-chemistry that interferes with the ability to filter out other realities while in this reality. The result is a garbled reality here, coupled with a tendency to visit other realities, some of which have very different basic assumptions and laws of perception. We could learn much about consciousness if we could get past our diagnostic prejudices.

Alcoholism is usually an addiction to sugar and thus, it is absolutely necessary to eliminate sugar as well as many carbohydrates. Supplements include a good amino acid capsule containing the full set of aminos, the B-vitamins, especially Vitamin B-3 in the niacinamide form, a good multiple-vitamin/multiple-mineral capsule, extra zinc, Vitamins A and C, chromium to help regulate blood sugar, manganese, milk thistle to repair the liver, and flaxseed oil or hempseed oil to supply Omega 3

---

[89] Read *Nutrition and Mental Illness* by Carl Pfeiffer PhD, MD, Healing Arts Press, Rochester, VT, 1987, for an eye-opening look at nutrition and its effect on mental illness.

and 6. The Liver Flush is very important here, as is walking and stretching on a regular basis.

As children, many alcoholics and drug addicts made very poor decisions about themselves and life. Often, these old decisions have not been examined, updated, or re-made in the light of adult information and consciousness. Specific forms of guided imagery have proven to be startlingly powerful in healing the emotional pain of alcoholics and can result in an 80% rate of rescission among alcoholics, something almost unheard of in most drug and alcohol counseling centers. [90]

Aggressive, autistic, or ADHD children almost always have calcium and magnesium deficits, are low in Vitamin B-6, and have heavy metals in their brain and blood, and thus, suffer from neurotoxicity. A number are also allergic to the food in their diet – especially sugar. Neither are they getting enough of the necessary fats. Often, they have a sluggish liver and colon, and are not getting the full range of vitamins and minerals they need because of poor absorption. Through chelation, plenty of outdoor play and exercise, whole foods, a good supply of the saturated and superunsaturated fats, as well as a steady supply of nutrient-dense foods, supplements, and enzymes, even cases of autism are being reversed completely. [91]

Exercise

Notice that all of the above healing programs utilize exercise and/or active physical play. Physical movement in the form of exercise is essential to the success of any healing program. I recommend getting a copy of the book *The Ancient Secret of The Fountain of Youth* and doing the five exercises described in it on a regular basis.[92] These exercises are basic to a healing program. I have been doing them for 20 years and have found them to be invaluable because they help keep the endocrine system in good working order, which is needed to run the body smoothly and well and to slow down the aging process.

---

[90] Michael Hutchinson, *Megabrain Report* (Sausalito, CA: Megabrain Inc, Vol. 1, Number 3 and 4).
[91] A Guiding Light in Nutritional Intervention in *The PPNF Journal*, Price-Pottenger Nutrition Foundation, LaMesa, CA, Spring 2000, Vol. 24, No. 1.
[92] Peter Kelder, *The Ancient Secret of the Fountain of Youth* (New York, NY: Doubleday, 1998).

I love these five exercises because they take only 15 minutes to do, and they are extremely powerful. They keep the core muscles of the body in good shape, keep the body flexible, eliminate fatigue, and produce a huge amount of energy, which lasts for approximately 60 hours – over two days! They also eliminate cellulite from thighs and arms, tighten sagging jowls, keep the bladder from leaking, clear sinus passages, reduce headaches, keep the neck flexible, and restore strength to the upper body in the shoulders, arms, wrists, and hands.

It is a good idea to get a few weights and lift weights a couple of times a week because weight-bearing exercise keeps your bones strong. You don't have to bench-press 200 lbs.! Just lift 5 lbs. with each arm or leg a dozen times or so and that is enough.

A wonderful tool for maintaining good health is a rebounder, which is something like a small trampoline. You stand on it and bounce lightly up and down, which helps drain tissues and clear the lymph system.

I recommend getting at least one exercise video, perhaps a beginning yoga routine, then using it at least once or twice a week as an alternate set of movements. And walk. Go outside and walk briskly, swinging your arms and taking big strides. Jog a little now and then. Run a little if you feel like it. Breathe deeply. Allow yourself to sweat. Above all, try to reclaim some of the huge range of movement and motion you enjoyed as a child.

Inner Work to Change Yourself

Excellent nutrition goes a very long way toward creating a balanced mind that matures beautifully into a wise, tolerant, peaceful personality. Yet it cannot make up entirely for poor child-raising practices, education that teaches competition rather than cooperation, or a socio-cultural system that promotes victimhood and the "every man for himself" approach to living.

Be aware that every behavior is accompanied by a feeling to which we have assigned a specific meaning. Many of these assigned meanings are contradictory from family to family or culture to culture. This results in a great deal of confusion and miscommunication. Some well-known examples of this are that in some cultures (American), you are taught to feel good if people respect your personal space "bubble" and stay an arm's length away when talking. In other cultures (Middle

Eastern), you are taught to feel insulted if someone remains an arm's length away. In some cultures (American), you are taught that it is okay to clean your teeth with a toothpick after meals and it is not okay to pick your nose. In other cultures (Thailand), people are taught that it is the grossest of habits to pick one's teeth, yet it is perfectly acceptable to pick your nose in public. In some families, it is acceptable to openly discuss one's finances or one's age, whereas in others it is considered the height of rudeness to bring up such subjects. In some families, it is okay to use sarcasm as humor, to stand up to others to the point of bullying them, or to use alcohol freely. In other families, sarcasm is considered a slap in the face, pushing one's own ideas forward is considered argumentative, and alcohol is an escape.

In addition to the stress that results from learned prejudices and biases, there are dozens of conditions in the body that result in bad moods, poor attitude, slow cognition, or mental and emotional fatigue. Some of the more common are PMS, low thyroid function, chronic fatigue syndrome, heavy metal toxicity, and disruption of the endocrine system by exposure to fungicides, pesticides, or other chemicals. Although these moods and attitudes are a problem for some, the bigger problem is that too many people are not self-aware and do not realize they don't have to feel the way they do.

When you are faced with the need to heal yourself, spend time examining *why* you think and feel the way you do. Get support from a counselor, coach, or therapist who will help you change habitual patterns of thinking and responses that have proved to be destructive or that no longer work for you.

With good nutrition, some detox, a bit of exercise, less stress, more rest, time for oneself, a little support, and some common sense therapy, life can be much sweeter and more peaceful.

High-nutrition foods are necessary if you want to maintain a life of restfulness, calm insight, dynamic creativity, and a peaceful demeanor. When the diet is nutrient-poor, you will not be able to produce the internal biochemistry and neurotransmitters that allow you to experience good moods while avoiding perceptual confusion, mental difficulties, and depression. ❖

25
Thinking ourselves well...

FEW THINGS ARE MORE IMPORTANT to you and your quality of life than high-nutrition food on a consistent basis. Few things are more detrimental to you than manufactured food filled with sugars and chemicals and lacking in nutrition.

A decade ago when I was working as an educational consultant, a couple of men came to visit me one day. One was head of a learning program for gifted children in Warren, Michigan. The other was the principal of a Lansing-area school. As we talked, I discovered that the principal's wife had cancer and was struggling terribly with the disease.

Knowing that I was into New Age thinking and believed in alternative health, the principal asked me if there was anything I knew of that might help his wife. Not really knowing what to say, I handed him a popular platitude of the times, "Well...you know, she must want that experience, and you should ask her why she created that disease for herself..." The implication being that she could just think otherwise and she would be well again.

Almost explosively he interrupted me. "Oh god! Don't ever say that to her. She's heard that over and over, and her response is, 'I don't *want* this damned disease, I *never* wanted this damned disease, and don't try to tell me that I did! No one ever wants cancer, and no one in their right

205

mind would ever create such a nightmare for themselves, so don't tell me I created it! That's bull----!'"

After he left, I thought deeply about what had been said. I had to agree with his wife. No one in her right mind ever wants cancer, even unconsciously. I wouldn't want it, and I could see how his wife would feel outraged when offered such a cheap answer. She was beyond the shallow excuses of most New Age thinking and needed something real, something she could trust to guide her toward healing.

I loved the whole New Age movement because it was a refreshing change of pace that made room for more of my humanity. Yet in that moment, it came up short. The whole movement looked like the emperor without any clothes, and it was at this moment that I discovered the difference between *believing* in something and the *knowing* that comes from real experience with something. Fluffy-sounding, sophisticated platitudes were useless. The woman was dealing with cancer. Her life was on the line. Where was the core of information and solid experience that would lead to something constructive, in this case, health and life?

This little episode made a big impression on me, one I've never forgotten. However, it was years before I could address the implication that we could just think ourselves well. One day the question I had posed to the principal revised itself from "W*hy* did she want to create that disease for herself...?" to the question "H*ow* did she create that disease...?"

Suddenly, there was the answer. *Of course* she didn't want the disease! She wanted to be healthy. But perhaps she also wanted to eat a lot of sweets...maybe she was too busy and on the run to find and prepare excellent meals...maybe she hated to deal with food at all...maybe she didn't believe in taking supplements...maybe she was being swept up in the pressures and politics of her husband's school district and had been living in a state of stress for years...perhaps she was struggling with a child or aging parent and didn't realize that time for herself was critically necessary...maybe she didn't realize the importance of avoiding pesticides, heavy metals, and all the other toxins that were being sprayed on our foods. Wanting all of these things and wanting good health amounted to wanting contradictory things.

If we *think* we can eat foods with no nutrition in them...if we *think* we can spray pesticides and other extremely poisonous chemicals on our foods...if we *think* we can manufacture food instead of eating the foods Nature has produced for us to eat...if we *think* we can lead lives of great stress and dismiss that stress as a mere emotional figment...if we *think* we can cover up the early warning signs of physical degeneration with drugs...then we are going to end up creating nightmarish diseases that we will have to deal with or die. It is in this way that we can think ourselves ill or think ourselves well. We do create our reality with our minds, and then we act accordingly.

The principal's wife may have been caught in the gap created by wanting contradictory things. All too often, we live an unexamined life dictated by forces outside ourselves. Life in America seems to be organized around the concepts of "grow up, get an education, get a job, get married, buy the best and biggest house you can afford, establish a nuclear family, work hard to make as much money as possible, collect as many symbols of the good life as you can, retire, and travel before you die."

What I am suggesting in this book is that we organize ourselves around a different set of concepts. They are similar, yet powerfully different. They are: grow to full maturity, commit to personal growth and the development of your natural potentials, learn to feed yourself, learn to educate yourself, learn to heal yourself, find work you like and be disciplined enough to figure out how to live while doing that work, organize your work and home life to maintain balance and health, marry if you can find someone who is as committed to your own development as their own, find a group of people you can live and work with and invest there to create a family of small businesses that all complement one another, think twice – no, three times – before having a child, work in such a way that you contribute to, support, and are celebrated by the entire family of people and businesses you are part of, learn to enjoy your work as much as possible (even the parts you do not care for as much), age wisely allowing your work to change as you do, give up the idea of death, travel only when absolutely necessary, and communicate with people and the world on an ongoing basis. [93]

It has been my experience that *if you really want to heal yourself, you have to heal your whole life.* You can do some of this healing yourself, and some can be done by others who help you. The most important factor in whether you get well or not is whether you begin a healing program or not.

Thousands of people don't feel good on a regular basis, but the doctor cannot find anything wrong with them. This does not mean they are healthy. You should be aware that by law, an allopathic doctor cannot treat

---

[93] See my book, *Robes: A Book Of Coming Changes,* for views of the future that may inspire you.

you for anything until something is clearly and obviously wrong. The rules of current medicine require the doctor to send you home and wait until a condition develops to the stage where he or she can diagnose it with current medical tests, then treat it with common drugs or surgical procedures. This is tragic because things should not have to get critically bad in the body before you do something. However, for a doctor to do otherwise is to open himself and his practice to being disciplined by the hospital he is connected to or being rejected by the insurance company because the treatments don't arise from a clearly defined and delimited diagnostic procedure. By delaying diagnosis and action, the doctor satisfies the requirements of the medical world he works in, yet opens him- or herself to being sued for not taking action much earlier. The problem is not with the doctor, it is with a system that demands a clearly defined disease to which a host of standard medical procedures can be applied.

It is too bad that our current medical system evolved into such a rigid creature because it truly hogties our physicians. They are not encouraged to learn about nutrition, herbs, detox, or natural therapies, many of which allow for full healing in very early stages of disease or illness. Instead, they are forced to wait until there is a disaster or an emergency. I know that things are changing, but it's oh so slowly.

In the meantime, make your health a high priority and take the steps you can to keep yourself in good health. When you have to see a medical doctor, choose one with the idea that you are selecting a partner who must work *with* you, not *on* you, and find one who is aware of the power of nutrition, detox, herbs, and exercise. For most of us, it is not a choice of either/or…either allopathic medicine or alternative and holistic medicine. Think in terms of sustainable, complementary medicine. Sustainable medicine does not do as much or more damage than it does healing. And complementary medicine requires deciding what you need from all sides of the various healing traditions – allopathic included – then knowing how to mix and match or blend drugs, herbs, foods, surgeries, exercise, and the many healing practices that are our heritage at this point in time.

While you are healing the body and changing your physical routines to those that support and nurture life, consider healing your heart, your mind, your house, your clothing, your room arrangements, your relationships, your perceptions, your work, and the earth. Start now with something small. Continue each day with another step. In time, you will be healed. When you are, it will feel like the world is a wonderful, beautiful place. It is…and that is how it should be. ❖

Part 6
Healing Techniques and Sample Programs

26
Tools and Techniques Used In Natural Healing

IF THERE IS ANYTHING to be aware of as you look through this section of the book, it is that all of the procedures described here call for you to not only be involved in your own healing processes, but to also give yourself permission to take the time you need for yourself and your healing.

For you to get sick, it takes time and a willingness to ignore the signs and symptoms of approaching disease. For you to heal, it takes time and the willingness to learn, to become more aware, to pay attention to what you are doing to yourself, and to do the things that support and nurture the body. If your ill health has become a way of life for you, then returning to good health requires that you develop an entirely new way of living. This is a tall order, but well worth the effort. The suggestions in this chapter are certainly not all that can be done, but they will get you started.

Castor Oil Pack

For many problems, it's hard to beat the pain-relieving and restorative power of a castor oil pack. This is an old Edgar Cayce remedy that is worth its weight in gold. It can be used regularly for every kind of healing from asthma, arthritis, and PMS to colds, cancers, infections, and ulcers. Not only does it help draw toxins from the body, the oil itself contains nutrients that nourish tissues and structures.

To make a castor oil pack you will need:

> About ¼ yard of wool flannel or cotton flannel fabric
>
> 16 oz of cold-pressed castor oil (Home Health is the Edgar Cayce brand)
>
> A piece of plastic about 12" by 15"
>
> A bath towel and a hand towel
>
> A heating pad
>
> 8 oz of water and a good book

1. To get the many benefits of a castor oil pack, you will need to use the pack **2 hours a day for 5 days in a row, then take 3 days off, then use it again, 2 hours a day for 5 more days in a row.**

2. To make the pack, fold and trim the flannel so that you have a rectangle of fabric that is **four-layers of fabric thick and about 9" by 12" in size.** Cayce recommended wool flannel but I use cotton flannel because I am so allergic to wool.

3. Next, get a plastic bag or piece of old shower curtain and **cut a piece of plastic that is about 12" by 15".** It should be larger than the flannel piece by about 2 inches on all sides, and if you're a squirmy, wiggly kind of person who has difficulty sitting still, the piece of plastic should be even bigger in case it shifts and gets out of place. Of course, if you're truly resting, the plastic should stay in place easily!

4. Lay the folded flannel on the plastic. **Open the castor oil and drizzle it in a thin stream back and forth over the flannel.** Let that soak in for a few minutes, then add more castor oil and let that soak in. Continue this process until all four layers of the flannel are saturated with castor oil. It should be damp but *not* dripping, or later, you'll have oil everywhere once the oil warms up and gets runny. A 9" by 12" pack of cotton flannel will use about 8-10 oz of the castor oil. I'm not sure what amount the wool flannel would use, probably less. When the pack is saturated, fold both the flannel and the plastic in half, so that the flannel is inside the plastic. Your pack is now ready to heat.

5. Pick a spot to sit or lay down, and **lay out the bath towel so that it will be under you to protect the chair or bed in case the oil runs.** Make sure you can also **plug in the heating pad** in that location.

Once the heating pad is plugged in, turn it on "medium heat." Fold the heating pad in half, putting the folded castor oil pack in between the halves of the folded heating pad. Allow to warm for 3-5 minutes.

6. While the pack is warming, **get a hand towel, an 8 oz glass of water, a good book** or magazine (or the TV remote control) and put them within reach of the place where you will be sitting or laying down.

7. Meanwhile, **get undressed.** If you are going to put the pack on your chest (for colds, asthma, bronchitis, pneumonia, heart trouble, breast tumors, infection, injury, etc.), you need to undress from the waist up. If it is winter, wear a loose robe so that your arms and shoulders will stay warm once the pack is in place. If you are going to put it on your abdomen (for immune system stimulation, cramps, gastrointestinal difficulties, hip problems, PMS, tumors, surgical incisions, infection, or injury, etc.), you will have to undress from the waist down. Have a blanket or afghan available to put over your tummy and legs so you won't get chilled. You can also put the pack on a leg or foot, on your upper back and neck, on your lower back, your arm or hand, or wherever you have pain or difficulty.

8. When the pack is no longer chilly, unfold the heating pad and take out the castor oil pack. Unfold the castor oil pack to its full size of 9" by 12" and **place the oil-saturated flannel against your chest** (or back, abdomen, leg, etc.). Next, **place the piece of plastic over the oil-soaked flannel** to prevent oil from getting on other clothing or the heating pad. **Put a hand towel over the plastic** to absorb any oil that may seep out if the plastic and flannel get out of alignment. You can also wear an old t-shirt instead of the towel, and this will keep your arms and shoulders covered if the room is cool.

9. Sit down (or lay down) and **put the heating pad over the hand towel.** You now have a stack of items that goes – from the bottom up – your skin, the oil-saturated flannel, the plastic protection, a hand towel, and the heating pad. Arrange your robe or afghan over all this so you are comfortable and then **sit and relax for two hours** while the castor oil soaks into your body through the skin and goes to work. You can read, take a nap, watch television, knit or do other needlework, draw, write letters, or just think and daydream.

10. **Drink the water when you are half way through the time.** If you drink it too soon, you may end up having to get up and go to the bathroom, which can be a nuisance because you end up trying to hold the

pack and plastic and towel in place while moving about, getting to the toilet, etc.

11. **When the two hours are up, remove the pack from your skin,** folding it in half so that the oil-soaked flannel is inside the plastic.

12. Use a paper towel to blot up some of the oil on your skin, then **wash the remaining oil off with a warm, soapy washcloth,** rinse, and pat dry. This is to make sure that you don't develop any allergies to castor oil. It is a powerful healing agent and one that you want to be able to use whenever you need it. **After this, you are finished** and free to go on and do whatever you like with the rest of your day or evening.

Store the castor oil pack in a cool, dark, dry place. It will keep well for six months and can be used again and again during that time. You may have to add a bit more oil if you use it a lot over a period of time and your skin has sucked most of the oil out of the pack.

If you live in a warm, moist climate, store the pack in the refrigerator or it will get moldy. I store mine in the refrigerator as a general practice in all seasons. Each person should have their own pack and use it for about six months before getting new flannel and making a new one. Depending on what you're trying to heal, you may have to make a new pack every month or perhaps only once a year.

I have seen some wonderful improvements using the castor oil pack. Some people notice a significant improvement in just the first one or two days. If this happens for you, don't stop using the pack until the entire thirteen days (5+3+5 days) is up. All kinds of secondary benefits and strengthening of the immune system take place during that time.

Mustard/Cayenne Foot Soak

Sometimes called the "mustard foot soak," this particular detox procedure is very helpful for headaches, the muscle aches and pains of colds and flu, water retention in the ankles or other parts of the body due to arthritis, diabetes, gout, poor circulation, and heart trouble, or the overall "blahs and goopiness" that accompany fasting, dieting, infections, and cancers or their treatments – chemotherapy, surgery, or antibiotics.

Your feet are a major outlet for toxic waste and since many people have such poor circulation in their legs, the feet become a storage site for waste instead of an outlet. The combination of warm water plus the healing properties of mustard and cayenne serve to both increase circulation and draw toxic waste right out through the feet.

To do this simple but powerful procedure...

1. You will need **a towel** and **a dishpan** or **basin of very warm water.** One of those foot-soaking appliances sold at the drug store works very nicely as well. The water should be deep enough to cover your feet without overflowing the pan when you put your feet in.

2. Add one tablespoon **(1 TBSP) of powdered dry mustard** and one teaspoon **(1 tsp) of cayenne pepper** to the water. Stir briefly just to distribute these two herbs.

3. Sit in a comfortable chair and **soak your feet in the basin for 30-40 minutes.** When finished, dry your feet with the towel and dump out the water, since it should not be re-used. **And that's it, you're done.**

The mustard soaks can be repeated 2-3 times a day and should be continued at least daily during periods of intense toxicity when the body is getting rid of a lot of waste, old cells, and metabolic structures that the body is breaking down because they are diseased or of poor quality construction. As you soak your feet, you will feel the intense heat of the mustard and cayenne working on your feet and legs. Even if the water cools off a bit, you will still feel the heat of these two herbs, and you will continue to feel them for several hours after you are finished with the soak.

Many people have thick, crusty skin on their feet or a variety of corns and calluses. These are the result of poor circulation and lack of care of the feet. In addition to the poor circulation mentioned above, there can be poor bone and tendon construction that started right from birth or as the result of bad or absent nutrition, badly fitting shoes, poor choice of shoes, being on one's feet for long hours every day, injuries that didn't heal correctly, and many other difficulties. If you begin doing mustard/cayenne foot soaks, you have an opportunity to soak and scrape away much of this thickened skin, which interferes with your ability to eliminate toxins through your feet.

I often encourage people to take a very dull knife, one that is *not* serrated, and, using a flat, scraping motion, scrape the sides, heels, toes, tops, and bottoms of the feet to remove dead, thickened skin on the feet. You can also use a loofa sponge, a nylon "scrubbie," or a pumice stone, but they don't work as well as the knife. The loofa or scrubbie are fairly difficult to clean and can become so smelly after a few days that you won't want to touch them!

Even if you only do one mustard/cayenne foot soak, you will feel light on your feet afterwards. If you do them daily, there will be less pain in your feet and legs, less swelling, more healing of sores and tender spots, and even easier breathing and better clarity of mind, all because of the improved circulation and reduction of toxic waste inside the body.

I buy dry mustard and cayenne in bulk form, at least a pint of each at a time and sometimes more, from our local health food store. You can also get them from your regular grocery store, but they come in tiny amounts. You end up having to pay for all the little bottles or cans, which you then have to throw away. If you don't have a good natural food or health food store nearby, however, what's available at the grocery store will get you started.

The Salt and Soda Bath

A salt and soda bath can be used by almost anyone trying to recover from almost anything, and it is most powerful for those trying to heal the more challenging problems like cancer or tuberculosis, AIDS, MS, lupus, hepatitis, fibromyalgia, drug addiction, or depression.

You should do a salt and soda bath when you are feeling your worst. It is during these periods of most intense toxicity that this bath shines! The baking soda and salt help to get toxins moving and released through the skin. This bath is especially helpful when you are nauseous, coughing, in pain, severely fatigued or unable to think and focus because of general irritability and restlessness. It is also very good for any sores on your skin.

To do a salt and soda bath...

1. **Run a bathtub full of very warm water**.

2. While the water is running **add one cup (1 c) of baking soda (sodium bicarbonate) and one cup (1 c) of salt** to the tub. The salt can be sea salt, real salt, natural salt, kosher salt, or if nothing else is available, regular table salt.

3. **Get in the tub and lie down** with as much of the body submerged as possible for at least **20 to 30 minutes,** although 45 minutes would be better. Add water if it gets too cool.

4. When finished, get up, **dry yourself by moving the towel slowly and with very firm pressure over your skin to remove as much dead skin as possible.** Then get dressed and **you're done**.

Do not put any lotions or oils on your skin for 24 hours, as these greatly reduce your body's ability to release toxic gases and wastes through the skin. It also interferes with the air available to skin cells, and if the lotion itself is full of toxins, it ends up putting back into the skin what you have just tried to remove.

If you are seriously ill, do a salt and soda bath every day until the nausea, weakness, fatigue, headaches, muscles aches, or other symptoms have diminished. The fact that your symptoms diminish usually does not mean that you are completely healed, however, it does mean that your immune system is coping with the problem much better than it was before. True healing usually has to be completed by detox and the top-quality nutrition that supplies the body with what it needs to repair and rebuild all of its structures.

When you are completely healed, fatigue disappears and you will have a steady supply of high energy, creativity, good spirits, curiosity, a desire to return to work or to find work you truly love, a sense of strength, and inner peace. You will sleep well, enjoy exercise, care about what you eat, and take an interest in your world. If you do not have the energy to do these things, then you are not well, even if there are no overt symptoms. Fatigue, or lack of pep, is one of the earliest signs that your body is accumulating too much waste matter. To help draw toxins and waste out of the body, do a salt and soda bath regularly. This can be every day during a cold or flu or on the days you are doing one of the detox procedures. It can be once or twice a week for maintenance; right before, during, or just after menstruation; or any time that you are struggling with the symptoms generated by serious health problems.

Castor Oil, Aloe, and Honey Packs

If you have serious sores or ulcers on your skin, especially your feet, ankles, and legs, start your healing by drinking a gallon of water every day. Do the Colon Sweep for five days, followed by the salt and soda bath outlined above every day for one week. Then speed the healing of your skin using the following procedures.

1. On each of **the first two days of your salt and soda bath, rub castor oil on** *only the area of your skin that needs healing* after you have finished the bath. (It would actually work even better if you put castor oil on a compress and taped it over a sore or ulcerated area the day before you're going to take a salt and soda bath. Remove the compress

just before the salt and soda bath next day, then put a new oil compress on after the bath that day.)

2. On **the next five days of your salt and soda bath, when you are finished with the bath, put a good amount of honey on a gauze compress and put the compress on the sore or ulcerated area** that needs healing. Change the compress daily.

3. If the sore or ulcer is not healed by this time, **return to using the castor oil** for one week after soaking the affected area in water for at least ½ hour each day.

4. If the sore is not healed by this time, **alternate back to using the honey** again, and continue the daily soaks.

5. Continue to **alternate between castor oil and honey, with daily soaks, until full healing is accomplished**. Take your vitamins and minerals regularly. Consider doing a Liver Flush and Purge.

If you have a serious burn...

Begin with aloe vera for the first two days, or as soon as possible. Use *fresh* aloe vera, don't use something out of a bottle or jar.

1. Before you cut a piece from the aloe vera plant, take a minute to **touch the plant where you are going to make the cut and tell it you would like to use it to heal someone.** Then give the plant a few minutes to adjust itself. It will often mobilize its healing energies into the area you are going to cut so that the piece you cut off will do a good job for the person who needs healing. It also prepares itself to heal the wound that will be left behind once you remove a piece from the plant. While the plant is getting ready, get a sharp knife, a gauze compress, and some tape.

2. When you and the plant are both ready, **cut a piece from the plant** that is slightly longer than the burn or sore, if possible.

3. The next step is to **cut open the piece of aloe so that you can unfold it and make it lie flat against the skin**. To do this, take the knife and carefully pierce the top layer of aloe skin (without cutting all the way through), and slice down the piece of aloe lengthwise. You now have a piece of aloe with a slice down the center and two flaps, one on each side.

4. Take the knife and slide it along under the left flap of the lengthwise cut you just made. Repeat this on the right side.

Step 1-2.   Step 3.

Step 4.   Step 5.

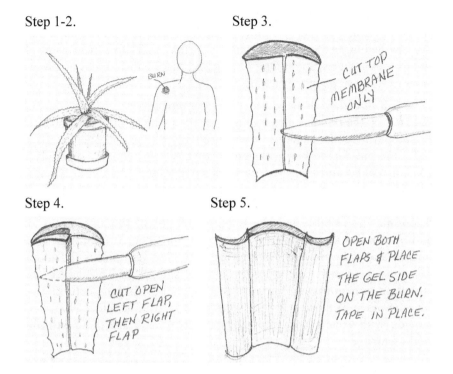

5. **Open up the piece of aloe, exposing the thick, meaty, juicy, gel-like interior and place this gel side directly on the burn.** If you need to cover a large area, cut two, three, or more pieces of aloe as described above and place them on the burn. If it is good aloe, you should be able to taste a slightly bitter taste in your mouth within five minutes of putting the aloe on your skin.

6. **Hold the aloe in place using a gauze compress** and tape. If the burn covers a very large area and the person is in bed, compresses and tape may not be practical. In this case, use something that is light in weight to hold it in place, like a folded towel. If the burn is on a leg or arm, use an ace bandage to hold the aloe pieces in place. **Leave the aloe in place for 12-24 hrs.**

7. **On day two**, (or after 12 hrs.), remove the compress, the weighted towel, or the ace bandage. Look at the aloe vera. All that should be left of the aloe vera will be a paper-thin piece of green plant skin lying on the burned area. **Remove this thin green skin carefully and replace with fresh aloe.** Cover or wrap as you did the day before, and **leave for another 12-24 hours**. Over these two days, your body

absorbs all of the aloe vera's thick, meaty interior and uses it to stop the burn from going deeper, to alleviate its heat, and to limit its damage. If you are healing a third-degree burn, you may want to repeat using the aloe pieces for Day 3 and Day 4, as noted below, then continue on with the rest of the steps in the healing

8. **On day three**, remove the compress, towel, or ace bandage and pick up the remains of the thin green aloe vera skin. If you had a first degree burn (reddened skin), it will probably be gone altogether. If you had a second-degree burn (blistered skin), the blisters will probably be gone, it will be much less red, perhaps smaller, and although it is seldom painful at this point, it will be tender, especially if it comes in contact with warm water. If you had a third degree burn (red, blistered, opened flesh), the flesh will usually be smooth and closed, although it may still be bright red with no skin over it. If the third degree burn area is not smooth and red, you may want to use new aloe vera pieces for another day or two. In any case, after the skin is smooth and bright red, it is important to **begin using honey** to feed the newly forming cells that will take the place of those cells that were destroyed in the burn. Honey will provide such excellent nutrition for the burned skin that there will often be no scarring.

9. Spread honey – raw is best but not necessary – in a thick layer on a compress that is large enough to cover the entire burn. **Put the honey compress on the burn** so that the honey is directly in contact with the burned area. **Leave it on for 24 hrs.**

10. **The next day**, lift the honey compress off the burn and put new honey on the compress. Or simply **replace it with a clean honey compress.**

11. **Repeat steps 9 and 10 every day until the burn is completely healed**, which is about 2-4 days for a first-degree burn, 4-6 days for a second-degree burn, and 5-14 days for a third-degree burn.

Note: If the burn is a 4th degree burn and very serious (the flesh is blackened and shrunken), or if it covers a very large area of the body, using large quantities of fresh aloe vera for more than a week can cause stomach cramping. If this happens, stop using the aloe vera and switch to honey for a few days. If the burns are extensive and severe, return to using aloe vera after a 3-5 day break, then alternate between aloe vera and honey until the healing is complete.

This method of healing burns often leaves no scars or discoloration of the skin. Sometimes the healing is so perfect you cannot tell there was ever a burn there. The fresh aloe vera is a natural antibiotic, and the honey is an even more powerful antibiotic, thus the biggest problem accompanying burns or any breach of the skin, which is secondary infection, is safely taken care of. If an infection gets started, use The Purge to end it.

Skin Brushing

One excellent way of cleaning and stimulating your lymph system, while also detoxifying your skin, is skin brushing. Although it seems almost too simple, it feels very good and is a very effective healing technique.

To do skin brushing...

1. You will need **a long-handled brush with natural vegetable bristles**. Synthetic, plastic bristles are often rough and can make tiny cuts in your skin, so be choosy in selecting a brush. Except for an occasional wash and rinse, the brush should be kept dry and used dry.

2. A good time to do skin brushing is first thing in the morning when you get up, *before* you take a shower or get dressed. You can also do skin brushing at night, just before you go to bed.

3. Your body should be dry, and you should move the brush over the skin in long sweeping motions – no back-and-forth or scrubbing motions. Imagine you are brushing toward the heart...up the legs, up the arms, down the neck, and up the trunk. It is not necessary to brush the face, but I do so occasionally just because it feels so good.

4. Skin brushing can be done once a day for maintenance, twice a day if you are under the weather, and can be increased to four times a day in periods of intense toxicity when dealing with the effects of problems such as cancer, AIDS, TB, pneumonia, weight loss miseries, all kinds of infections, or anything that makes you feel awful.

It only takes a few extra minutes to brush your skin and is a startlingly wonderful way to begin the day simply because you will feel so alive all over. It is also a great way to end the day because it leaves you calm and relaxed.

❖

Juicers and Juicing

When I first set out to heal myself, one of the prescriptions was a pint of carrot juice every day. The recommendation from Dr. Gonzales was to invest in a Champion juicer because it was, in his words, "a real workhorse, worth the money."

When I saw the price of the Champion, I balked. I did not want to put out $225 for a juicer. So I went to the store and came home with a nice looking juicer that cost $40. It lasted less than a week.

About that time, a friend offered to let me use his juicer – a $60 item – to do my juicing. That one lasted only two days, and I was back on the market looking for two juicers, one to replace his, and a good one with a decent motor for me.

An advertisement for a Vita Mix machine came in the mail just about then. After reading it carefully and swallowing hard at the $380 price, I sent for it because I wanted something that would do more than just juicing, and it had a sturdy motor. I was sure it would last more than a week even if used heavily. When it arrived, I plugged it in, put in my carrots, and ended up with carrot mush, a thick, mealy glob that was a long way from juice.

Hoping to salvage the situation, I got out some cheesecloth, thinking I would strain the juice out of the carrot cellulose and fiber. But the juice dripped out so slowly that, after half an hour, I only had half a cup of juice that was already turning bitter. My instructions from Dr. Gonzalez were to make a pint of juice and drink it immediately, before it oxidized, so I was beginning to feel desperate.

In an effort to get the juice out of the carrot mush, I tied the four corners of the cheesecloth in a knot to form something akin to a bag. Slipping a broom handle through the knot, I laid one end of the broom on the cupboard, put the other end on the back of a chair, and hung the cheesecloth full of carrot mush over a large pot on the floor. Then I started turning the cheesecloth bag in an attempt to squeeze the carrot juice out of the mush and extract the required juice quickly.

However, as the pressure built up in the cheesecloth bag, the juice began squirting in every direction, sometimes three or four feet across the kitchen. I ended up with carrot juice all over myself and the kitchen, ruined a good shirt with stains that wouldn't come out, had a colossal mess to clean up, and got barely a lick of juice. I needed something that would actually produce juice and had easy clean-up.

After looking around for a while, I came across someone at a conference demonstrating the Omega Juicer. This looked like the answer to my prayer. It was only $180, had a good motor, produced a very high quality juice, and was very easy to clean up via a thin paper filter that prevented fiber from getting into the blades or screens. You just put the paper filter into the juicer, made your juice, pulled the paper filter out with all the pulp attached, rinsed the machine, and you were done. I bought it.

The Omega worked wonderfully for me. It was quick and simple and easy to use. But when my husband went on the same healing program I was on, I discovered that I couldn't make the required amounts of carrot juice without stopping the machine, taking it all apart, removing the filter paper and pulp, putting in another filter paper, re-assembling the entire thing, and continuing on with the juice-making.

When a third family member got interested in healing, I began to run out of filter papers, had to keep ordering, and was tired of stopping to take the machine apart several times just to change the filter. I needed a juicer that was designed for continuous feed operation.

In the end, I bought the Champion. It had the powerful motor I needed, made excellent juice, allowed for continuous feed operation, didn't require the purchase of filters, and was extremely easy to clean up.

I still use the VitaMix because it makes great whole-fruit smoothies, as well as excellent fresh tomato juice, and a variety of creamed soups. I bought a citrus attachment for the Omega and use it to juice the oranges, lemons, and grapefruit needed for the Purge, and it does an excellent job of making fresh citrus juice drinks for breakfast. For my everyday carrot juice or any type of vegetable/fruit juice (celery, beet, apple, broccoli, cabbage, spinach, etc.), I use the Champion. Each of these machines does an excellent job at one aspect of juicing. My daughter, who has access to each of my juicers, decided to try a Juiceman II for her own kitchen. She says the Juiceman also does a very good job with vegetables and fruits, although she, too, uses the Omega for citrus juicing.

My original wish to avoid spending $225 on a Champion ended up costing me over $900 by the time I was finished. The lessons were, "Don't try to skimp by buying cheap, poorly built equipment" and "Know what the equipment will really do." By ignoring these two rules, you could end up spending more in the long run, and if using the equipment is such a hassle that you avoid doing what must be done, your healing efforts will be delayed, and you will suffer longer.

All of this is just to make you aware that to take charge of your healing, you will have to make a few investments in your kitchen equipment. A good juicer is one of those investments. Remember, fruit juices tend to break up wastes in the body, and vegetable juices tend to rebuild the body.

The gift of healing that comes with juicing is that you get all of the vitamins and minerals in the fruit or vegetable, but the body doesn't have to put forth any effort to extract them. When you drink a freshly made juice, the vitamins and minerals go directly into your system. Much of the body's work of digesting and breaking down the component parts of a plant in order to extract useful nutrients is eliminated. The burden on the pancreas to drop repair and rebuilding efforts and switch to the task of digestion is also avoided, and the valuable pancreatic enzymes that consume cancers and infectious organisms are free to continue their work of healing. The pancreas does not get worn out, and you do not degenerate in the steady downhill manner that is so common today.

Drinking only fresh, raw fruit or vegetable juices is one very powerful way to heal and rebuild. When you are unable to digest foods or too weak to eat, you can slowly, gently nourish your body back to health with raw fruit and vegetable juices.

Mineral Broths

In addition to juicing, making broth is a fabulous way to restore health and get high-density nutrition. When broth is made properly, you use bones from beef, pork, chicken, lamb, or fish, and all of the minerals that were used to build those bones are extracted and end up in the broth, which you then drink or use to make soup. This kind of broth or soup is very healing and can be made in quantity then frozen to be used later.

To make a good broth, put the following into a large stock pot:

> 3-5 lbs of beef bones. These can be raw or leftovers from a
>   roast. If making chicken broth I use chicken necks, backs,
>   and wings
> 5-8 quarts of water
> 1 large potato
> 2 large carrots
> 1-2 large onions

3 TBSP dried parsley or ½ cup fresh parsley

¼ cup of vinegar or red wine to acidify the water, which makes it possible to extract all the minerals from the bones

Simmer beef broth for 72 hours (3 days). Simmer chicken (or fish broth) for 36 hours. Strain everything out of the broth and do not re-use the vegetables. Add sea salt to taste, perhaps a little pepper, and it is ready to drink. If you are going to use some to make a soup, you may put cubed beef or chicken in the broth, add 1 TBSP of nutritional yeast, salt, fresh vegetables, and fresh or dried herbs such as 2-3 tsp of parsley, 1 tsp marjoram, basil or oregano. Simmer to cook vegetables, add ground pepper, and eat.

Raw Foods

There is nothing quite as drastic – or as powerful – as changing to a raw food diet. Cooked foods take a heavy toll on your health…an extremely heavy toll, all because the natural enzymes in the raw food that would help with digestion have been destroyed in the cooking process. Thus, I often tell people who need to do serious healing that raw foods are a major key to healing. Fruits, vegetables, grains, milk, eggs, butter, cheese, and even some organic meats can be eaten raw if you know how to prepare them.

Fruits and vegetables are easy – just wash and eat. Grains, as in 14-Grain Cereal, can be ground and soaked overnight. Raw milk may be illegal in your state, but can still be purchased if you can find a farm that sells shares of ownership in a cow. If you buy shares, then you have access to the raw milk, cream, and butter from that cow because it's your cow.

Raw eggs should be organic and can be eaten by making an eggnog drink as follows:

1 cup milk

1 raw egg

1 TBSP honey

1 dash nutmeg and/or cinnamon

Put all ingredients in a blender and blend until frothy. Sprinkle a little more nutmeg on top and drink. It's delicious and so good for you. Sometimes I will add strawberries, blueberries, peaches, yogurt, or hempseed oil to increase nutrition and add variety.

Raw cheese can be purchased at any good health food store. And raw meat should be *organic* liver that is cut in ½" cubes and frozen individually. Then, you take out 1or 2 frozen cubes, put it into a fruit smoothie, blend well, and drink immediately. I have seen this "smoothie-frozen liver" combination restore someone with fairly advanced multiple sclerosis to enough energy and health to set aside her wheelchair and heavy leg braces and return to walking.

I remember hearing long ago about people who were into raw foods, juicing, and a variety of other exotic practices like enemas, mineral baths, heavy exercise, and various forms of sweats. At the time, I thought they were just "health nuts" and wondered why anyone would bother with all that. Now I know…they were sick and had discovered the power of detox, raw foods, and the body's ability to heal itself if it was given complete support. In any healing program, raw foods, fresh vegetable and fruit juices, along with well-made mineral broths should be a mandatory part of your healing program.[94] [95]

If you're going to cook anything, make a good-quality broth. This, along with raw juices, brings healing and builds good, sturdy health.

At this point, several things bear repeating…If you are sick, change your diet. Start getting the high nutrition you need to rebuild. Exercise pushes nutrients into difficult-to-reach corners of the body; shoves waste materials out; promotes flexibility, strength, and energy; and allows organs to move around and stretch a bit within the tight confines of the body. Enemas, mineral baths, sweats, and specific detox procedures allow the body to return to youthful form and function, bring clarity, and zest for living.

Most people in first world countries are in terrible shape. Many are suffering from malnutrition. The first stage of malnutrition and starvation is a slightly swollen, puffy body. This puffiness then becomes a true overweight condition as people eat more than they should in an unconscious attempt to satisfy the body's need for nutrients. I hear people everywhere talking about trying to lose weight, or exhorting others to lose weight, or selling something to help people lose weight.

---

[94] To learn how to prepare excellent old-time foods, get *Nourishing Traditions* by Sally Fallon, ProMotion Publishing, San Diego, CA, 1995.
[95] Another great book full of raw food recipes is *Living Cuisine: The Art and Spirit of Raw Foods* by Renee Loux Underkoffler. It was published by Avery Publishing in 2003.

You cannot be suffering from low-level malnutrition and attempt to cut back on eating without disastrous effects, the least of which are depression, fatigue, and irritability. You may look nice and trim for a while, but without the input of high nutrition, you will go downhill and may end up triggering one of your genetic weaknesses. At the very least, you will feel crabby and hungry, and you may return to gorging yourself because you're so miserable.

I would suggest that, instead of just talking about our health problems or engaging in less-than-helpful efforts, we educate ourselves well and learn to recognize where the source of the real problem lies, then make the necessary changes in our lifestyles, food systems, and the world.

Herbs

There are so many good books already written about herbs, what to use, how to use them, the standard dosages required for a therapeutic effect, and the contra-indications to be aware of that I will not duplicate those efforts here. But I do have several things to say about the use of herbs.

The first is that herbs are powerful medicines. Everything you eat affects the body immediately. And anything that you take in a consistent manner – three times a day for more than two days in a row – is going to shift your biochemistry seriously, for better or for worse. Therefore, do not take herbs recklessly or without knowing their effects.

The second is that herbs you use should be grown here in the U.S. on an organic farm, or wildcrafted, otherwise you have no way of knowing whether pesticides like DDT or fungicides – banned here in the U.S. but still legal in foreign countries – have been used on them. Also, many imported herbs are irradiated before they are allowed into the U.S., and that destroys both the medicinal potency and leaves you taking in a substance whose energy fields have been seriously deranged.

The third is that, too often people take herbs in doses that are much too low because their potency has not been determined. Or the herbs they take are old, irradiated, or were poorly grown.

Many people try a few herbs and when nothing spectacular happens within a few days, they try something different. When you decide to take an herb, you must commit to taking it for at least three months as they work slowly and very gently. It won't usually take that long for you to notice improvements, but it might be helpful for you to understand that herbs work in terms of "getting to the source" of the problem. They start by correcting imbalances in the body and, like antibiotics, need to be taken for a certain period of time in order to do the whole job. They do not usually have unpleasant side effects, so at first you may not notice them working – but they are!

Often you should take an herb for three months and then stop for a couple of weeks, then resume for another three months. If you have a chronic problem, an herbal program can be repeated every year at the same time, as this allows the body to cope with the problem better.

Herbs are a perfect accompaniment to the exercise, detox, high nutrition diet, and supplement approach to healing. If herbs aren't working for you, it may be because you have too much waste matter in your body and you're too plugged up to absorb anything, or your circulation is so poor that nothing is reaching its destination, or your nutrition is so wretched that the effects of the herbs are overpowered. Clean yourself out, change your diet, and herbs will have a quick, powerful impact.

Clay Packs

I first heard about clay in the book *Secrets Of The Soil* by Peter Tompkins and Christopher Bird. The book noted that trees, plants, and animals whose water contained traces of montmorillonite clay had extraordinarily fine health, resistance to disease, and all sorts of other beneficial effects. Since I was aware that what is good for plants and trees is often good for humans, I immediately made note of the power of clay. [96]

Shortly after that, I read somewhere that the Indians of South America made small clay balls, dried them, and kept them in their pocket to swallow now and then, keeping their gastrointestinal tracts free of parasites, worms, and harmful bacteria.

When I came across a book called *Our Earth, Our Cure* by Frenchman Dr. Raymond Dextreit, [97] I started exploring the uses of clay in all sorts of situations in which people and animals required healing.

---

[96] Peter Tompkins and Christopher Bird, *Secrets of the Soil* (New York, NY: Harper & Row Publishers, 1989) p. 213-225.
[97] See Appendix B for a list of suggested references every home should have.

I put clay in the water our chickens drank, and they grew thick, shiny feathers while producing eggs with thick shells and bright orange yolks. I put clay in the cow's water and got rich, creamy, delicious milk and butter. I put clay in the dog's water and achieved some relief of her arthritis and a clearing up of her "dog breath." I put clay in the green-house beds and got healthy greens all winter, greens that froze again and again but then thawed out and kept growing, refusing to die. They eventually went to seed the following summer. Finally, I started taking a tablespoon of clay in a liquid suspension every morning and discovered that my hair and fingernails improved, I had less gas and bad breath, and enjoyed a general improvement in health overall.

When clay turned up as part of the Liver Flush in the detox program that was outlined by Dr. William Kelley and Dr. Nicholas Gonzales, the whole family adopted it.

Now I use clay for lots of things...on bee stings or bug bites; for small burns; for sores, acne, and ulcers – both internal and external; to stop bleeding; for nausea, diarrhea, or constipation; as a poultice to draw poisons and toxins out of the body; to reduce fevers and pain; help bring organs back to healthy functioning; to restore beauty, color, and texture to facial skin; and a host of other applications.

There are two kinds of clay you might hear about. One is Montmorillonite clay, the other is Bentonite clay. For all practical purposes, they are the same. I don't know who came up with the name Montmorillonite or when they came up with it, but the "Montmorillonite" moniker was fairly well-known and had been used for some time when another fellow named Benton came along, discovered a clay deposit, started mining it, and named his brand "Bentonite."

When it comes to application, I pay more attention to the color than the name. Green clay is the most potent, and I try to get green clay first. If I can't find green, I go for red clay. Other colors (gray, yellow, white, pink, brown, etc.) are also useful, but not quite as potent as green or red.

It is usually easy to find green or red clay in a small tube containing a few ounces of moist clay at your local health food store for around $8 per tube, but this is really expensive. I buy a 50 lb bag of powdered clay for about $16 from a local supplier and use it all year on people, plants, and animals.

To prepare the clay, put 2 cups of the dry clay in a glass or ceramic pot that has a cover. A covered casserole dish is a good "clay pot." So are the old-fashioned baked bean pots you can sometimes find at flea markets. Do **not** use plastic or metal to hold the clay, as clay will react with both of these materials, either turning the plastic to mush or absorbing some of the metal. Next, add clean water (distilled or reverse osmosis) that has not been boiled or treated in any way. Do not stir!

Let the clay sit without touching it until the water has been absorbed into the clay evenly. If necessary, add more water a little at a time. If it is too thin, add a little more dry clay to thicken it. Again, do not stir. When all the water has been absorbed and it looks as though it has a paste-like texture, put the cover on and leave it in a sunny place if possible. After a day, it is ready to use. To keep it from drying out and cracking, add a little water every week or so and let the water soak in slowly. It will keep for months.

For reasons that are not well understood, clay has the ability to draw toxins from everywhere in the body to the site where the clay poultice is sitting. Thus, if you have a leg ulcer due to diabetes, and you decide to use clay to heal the ulcer, it will pull all the toxins in your body to the area of the ulcer. This means the ulcer will get worse before it gets better. To avoid frightening yourself into thinking that you are getting worse or creating a more monstrous problem, it is helpful to eat only fresh fruits and salads for several days and take 1 TBSP of clay orally in the morning and in the evening before you begin applying a series of clay poultices.

My grandson, Kraig, is very allergic to mosquito and spider bites and any bite site tends to swell and become very red, sometimes reaching a diameter of two inches of angry, red skin that burns and itches for days, while he scratches and makes it all worse. One day, he had a particularly nasty bite, so we decided to apply clay to reduce the inflammation. Because he was only seven years old and fairly free of toxins – or so we thought – we didn't think fasting or a few days of oral clay was necessary, so we put the thick, clay poultice on his thigh, put a folded paper towel over it, wrapped the whole area with an ace bandage, and left it overnight.

The next day his entire leg was swollen and red! The day after that it was worse, taking on a dark red color. The clay had drawn all the toxins from his entire body into his thigh. It took nearly a week of clay poultices, warm baths, drinking lemon water (to fluidify the blood for better circulation), treatments with hot and cold water, and careful eating to bring the leg back to a normal state. A side benefit of using the clay was that, for a while, he was much less reactive to mosquito and spider bites because the clay had removed some of the toxic load his body had to deal with, leaving his immune system more able to deal with the small poisons deposited by mosquitoes and spiders when they bit him.

Getting Rid of Parasites

Parasites are an amazingly common visitor in the human body, and even if you do not have symptoms, you may have them. When I first went to see Dr. Gonzales and he said I had parasites, I was astounded. Now, I take a little bit of extra time every year to make sure I don't have them.

Since I live on a working farm, it is easy to pick up parasites in the warm summer months when I am outside a lot, walking barefoot. To help keep my gastrointestinal tract free of parasites, over the summer I regularly take a tablespoon of liquid Bentonite clay in the morning, followed by a ½ glass of warm water.

As autumn arrives and the year draws to a close, I buy a bottle of capsules called *Para Protect Factors* [98] and take 2 capsules at breakfast, lunch, dinner, and bedtime. That's 8 capsules a day for 6 days. There are 50 capsules in the bottle, so I will have used 48 of them after six days. On the morning of the seventh day, I take the remaining 2 capsules of *Para Protect Factors* and drink 3 cups of senna leaf tea over the rest of the day. Senna leaf increases bowel action, which helps to expel dead parasites. I do a set of coffee enemas as well, which helps clear the liver of any dead parasite material it filtered out of my blood.

Using Natural Products

If you are like I used to be, you probably don't give much thought to use of fancy, flavored, and perfumed items like toothpaste, deodorant, lotion, soap, or detergents. If you haven't given much thought to your toothpaste and toilet cleaner, it's quite likely you haven't even considered the sorts of things that are spread, dumped, or sprayed around your kitchen or onto your lawn. Perhaps you wouldn't think your house was clean if you didn't use powerful chemicals designed to kill everything on contact. And maybe you think your lawn would die or be ugly if you weren't spraying serious toxins and fertilizers on it.

---

[98] *Para Protect Factors* are made by Country Life. There are other herbal parasite remedies out there, this just happens to be the one I like.

You can't change your whole life, your mind, your habits, and perceptions overnight, but while I have your ear, I want to mention that once you get serious about healing and have gone through a detox program designed to remove toxins, you are going to begin noticing what you put in, on, or around your body. It's a slow-dawning awareness, but once begun, it continues. The most important thing for you to grasp at this point is that there are good, non-toxic substitutes for every commercial substance you currently use and a variety of alternate procedures for every process you are in the habit of performing. Our ancestors were not ignorant, suffering savages. In my opinion, they were practical, creative, observant, and even brilliant. They came up with a wide variety of solutions for every problem. Today, we are too dull and stressed to do this. We gape around for a one-size-fits-all, manufactured solution that we think we can afford.

To get beyond this, make yourself aware of "spincasting!" This is the ability of governments, corporations, and Madison Avenue to: 1. Spin a web of perception designed to make you believe what they want you to believe so you will either acquiesce to something, ignore something, or buy something; 2. Slant the facts just enough to create an attractive – but unbalanced and therefore unhealthy – view of someone, something, or some event; 3. Distract you with something interesting but irrelevant so that you will ignore the truth or fail to ask the really important questions.

The truth is that commercial toothpastes do not prevent cavities. The only thing that prevents cavities is a high nutrition diet. Toothpastes only cover the bad breath that often results from eating foods containing sugar. Rinsing the mouth with water or brushing with a dry toothbrush has as much power to deter cavities as brushing with toothpaste.

Most toothpastes have fluoride and sodium laureth sulfate in them, neither of which is good for you. In spite of the widespread perception that fluoride prevents cavities, the truth is that in the 1940s the government produced a lot of fluoride for the atomic bomb project. The fluorine gases emitted from these factories killed plants, trees, and sickened people and animals along the East Coast.

New Jersey area farmers who lost crops, cows, horses, and some family members sued. The government lost their case and eventually paid the survivors a very small sum of money (about $200) while hushing up the case. Looking for the perfect way to cover their need to continue producing fluoride for the Manhattan Project, the government suddenly declared that not only was fluoride harmless, it was good for you! In a perfect example of spincasting, they announced a decision to do some "research" and a few studies on fluoride because "it strengthened bones and teeth."

This was simply not true. In fact, the exact opposite was true. The research project gave the government an excuse to experiment and added an aura of legitimacy to fluoride use. It also allowed them to see how bad things could get when fluoride was introduced into the general population. They published a study that said fluoride was *not* harmful, and the men who worked in fluoride factories had fewer cavities. The actual truth was that most of these men had no teeth left because their teeth had been disintegrated by the fluoride fumes in the workplace! There was no mention either of the rubber boots the men had to wear because the nails in their leather boots kept disintegrating. [99]

Since the 1940s, other research has indicated that fluoride disrupts endocrine function, especially thyroid function. Fluoride in the water supply has been seriously implicated in Alzheimer's, Down's syndrome, autism, hip disorders, brittle bones, thyroid cancers, stiffness in joints, central nervous system effects, and a general drop in overall health and mental brightness, as well as mental and emotional stability. [100]

Here at the farm, my daughter makes all kinds of soaps and lotions that are wonderful and do not have any toxic products in them. I have a friend down the road who makes a tooth powder from salt, soda, orange peel, and sage. I love it, and it cleans my teeth a hundred times better than any commercial toothpaste. People sometimes ask, "...but what does the tooth powder taste like?", and I tell them it tastes fine, kind of salty with just a touch of soda.

Homemade tooth powders are different from commercial toothpaste in that they are usually not sweet, and they certainly have a different texture, neither of which is disagreeable. It only took me a couple of days of using the tooth powder to get to the point of definitely preferring it to toothpaste.

A good point to make here is that if you base every decision of what to eat or drink on whether something tastes good or not, you are

---

[99] "Fluoride, Teeth, and the Atomic Bomb," by Joel Griffiths and Chris Bryson; www.inter-view.net/~sherrell/bomb.htm, July, 1997. This page is no longer available on the Internet, but if you do a search for the authors' names, you will find other resources and information, including www.fluoridealert.org.
[100] "The Greatest 'Scientific' Fraud Yet?" *Nexus New Times*, Jan-Feb 2001, pg. 14-15.

using an immature system of judgment. This is like basing every decision on money. It simply doesn't work because the criterion is too narrow.

If your diet includes things like soda pop, candy, bottled or canned juice drinks, snacks, and processed foods containing sugars, you will be quite likely to reject anything that isn't based on sugar and doesn't taste sweet. This is disastrous for your body.

Changing your diet and eliminating sugar will allow your taste buds to normalize. If you do this for a few months, then go back to try your old diet for a day or two, you will be appalled at how thin and tasteless commercial foods are. You'll also be surprised at what a poor cleaning job regular toothpaste does. Then it will be easier to change to something that is good for you, including toothpaste.

As for deodorants, read the labels and you will find that a good many of them contain aluminum and aluminum compounds. Every time you put on deodorant in the morning, you are getting a dose of aluminum molecules. After a while, this can build up enough aluminum in your system to require chelation therapy. When added to the other heavy metals that you take in with your foods or in simply breathing, the effect on the body is deadly.

Do not use deodorants full of perfumes and chemicals or that are designed to inhibit wetness. There is nothing wrong with sweating; it is an important way of detoxing the body. Get a crystal stone from your health food store, wet it, and rub it over your armpits each morning. It prevents the growth of bacteria in your sweat and does not have harmful side effects. An added benefit is that you buy one stone for about $8, but it lasts two or three years, which is a tremendous savings. In addition, you are not buying the plastic cases or metal and plastic cans that many deodorants come packaged in, so you are reducing landfill wastes and ecological resources.

If you change your diet to whole food and eliminate white flour and white sugar, you will notice that your breath and sweat are much sweeter and your feet do not smell. Soon you'll become aware that many common products are designed and sold to cover up our poor physical condition. Most of them are marketed as if they will bring a sense of richness and luxury to your life, adding this illusion to the illusion of health and beauty.

Commercial shampoos are another illusion of luxury. They cost a fortune, yet most contain alcohol. Alcohol destroys hair follicles on your head and results in loss of hair. Many shampoos and bar soaps contain sodium laurel sulfate or sodium laureth sulfate, which create lots of foamy bubbles but are toxic.

When my daughter expressed an interest in making soaps and shampoos, I encouraged her. The soaps were wonderful but the shampoos left our hair with a thick, sticky build-up. To remove this build-up, we started rinsing our hair with vinegar until the hair squeaked. The results of using this odd combo were surprising. My hair, which is very fine and frizzy, had extraordinary body and still looked good after three or four days without shampooing. There was also much less hair loss on a daily basis. The norm for loss of hair is about 100 hairs per day. While I don't get down to counting actual hairs, I was surprised to notice that I was hardly losing any hair at all!

With commercial shampoos and conditioners, even the herbal kinds from health food stores, I had to wash my hair every other day or it looked flat and felt awful. Being able to stretch this to three days, or even four if I didn't have to go anywhere, and still look quite decent was a real bonus. Another benefit was less breakage and the disappearance of split ends. The bottom line for soaps and shampoos is to avoid commercial, synthetically perfumed products as much as possible. If you don't know someone who makes soap, get something as benign as possible from the health food store. After detox and a good supplement regimen, your itchy, scaly, patchy skin and scalp may clear up, and with natural products you may have far fewer allergies simply because you are not constantly exposing yourself to the chemicals used in so many common products.

There was a time when my cupboards were stocked with anti-bacterial soaps and detergents, bleaches, acids for dissolving limestone blotches around faucets, oven cleaners, spray polishes for furniture, cleaners and polishes for cooking pots, shower cleaners, floor disinfectants, water softeners, dryer sheets to prevent static cling, and a half-dozen other chemicalized items that I thought were necessary for any decently run home.

One day, I met a woman with breast cancer. She had come to visit the farm after reading one of my other books. For reasons I can't recall now, we ended up trading services, and to fulfill her part she wanted to do some housekeeping. I agreed, and we made the trade. When she went to work cleaning, she ignored all my expensive chemicals and asked if I had some vinegar, some baking soda, and a little dish soap for sensitive hands. I retrieved a bit of each requested substance from the kitchen, and she went to work, slowly and lovingly cleaning each guestroom.

I learned that day that my own cleaning style was crazy. I resembled a frenzied scrubwoman who spent most of the time holding her breath while running in and out of rooms so she wouldn't breathe in the chemicals she was spraying and splashing all over. I switched to simpler cleaning products and began to realize that the most powerful substance of all was just plain water.

Don't use powerful cleaning products that tell you right on their labels that you shouldn't get them on your skin or breathe in their vapors. They aren't necessary. How are you going to get anything done if you can't breathe? And when you think about it, it's a bit insane to use them in the first place. If the world were that dangerous and infectious a place, we would never have made it past caveman stage. As it is, half of us are suffering from the curse of Louie Pasteur who believed in the "war model" of bacteria-against-humans. The rest of us are suffering from the marketing myopia spread by those who specialize in advertising and marketing and who keep telling us what we need to buy/have/do.

The simplest products work merely by shifting the pH balance, thus making an inhospitable environment for bacteria. You don't have to kill bacteria, and in fact, you can't kill them. You only kill the weaker strains, as well as the beneficial bacteria, leaving the more virulent strains to multiply without restraint or limits. When the beneficial bacteria and weaker strains are left in place, they compete with the more virulent strains for nutrients and space, thus providing an effective means of controlling these more vicious forms. And with a healthy immune system, bacteria are not a threat. After all, we survived very well without commercial chemical products – whether for cleaning, antibiotics, or personal hygiene – for thousands of years.

The simple cleaning products such as soap and water, baking soda, vinegar, and even hydrogen peroxide are easy on your body, your pocketbook, and the environment. Once you stop believing that the expensive Madison-Avenue chemicals are part of the American Way, or begin to discover how destructive the American Way is, you will begin to wonder how you ever got so paranoid about using certain products. ❖

27
Sample Healing Programs

THIS CHAPTER CONTAINS a few samples of healing programs that I have used for various problems. Each program is meant to give you an idea of how to use the tools in your toolbox that I have talked about in earlier pages. Your tools are: food, exercise, detox routines, supplements, and special procedures such as baths and soaks, Castor Oil Packs, or other techniques. By combining these major cornerstones of all true healing, you can create a healing program for yourself or someone you love. Keep in mind as you read through these that every individual has to be considered through a unique lens. What heals one might be death for another. What one person tolerates easily, another is stressed beyond any useful point.

As you look through these programs, become aware of something called "healer's lag." This is a tendency to enter into a brief period of shock or delay in beginning a healing program. This lag often occurs because illness, even a slight fall-off in your health, affects perception immediately. You may not recognize the need to take action, or you may be unable to decide what to do. More often, people become frightened and don't want to deal with anything difficult. Yet, true healing requires you to *think and act on your own behalf.* You must *do something different* today if you want to feel better tomorrow. You might also have to take time away from work in order to really heal. Oddly, many people want to be healthy, but they don't want to heal themselves. They want someone else to do it for them or at least to *make* them do it. This gives them the feeling that someone cares about them.

Over the last 30 years, Americans have gotten into the habit of ignoring how they feel until they collapse. They pop a few pills while they continue to run to work, to social events, and a dozen other places. In their mind, the pill is doing the healing, and thus nothing more need be done. This is dangerous because the pills are merely covering up the body's warning signs, and if we are to become a healthy, viable nation once more, this idea must be replaced with the truth: the body is doing the healing and must be supported in its efforts.

If you subscribe to the ways of modern chemical medicine and take a pill that only suppresses symptoms while allowing you to keep going at full speed without changing, you are going to get worse, not better. The little flags that the body raises must be taken seriously and corrections made, or there will be a serious disease, usually within a couple of months, sometimes a couple of years. Then, instead of a few alterations in day-to-day living, you may need major surgeries, extended time off work, expensive tests and medicines, and who knows what else.

If you are tired of your job, feel trapped in dull, dead relationships, or want to do something else with your life but are afraid to change, the idea of being diagnosed with a major disease, having time off, and perhaps even going on permanent disability may seem attractive at first. It allows you to do something different. However, playing the role of "sickie" gets just as boring as a bad job or a dull spouse. If you get stuck in the limited incomes of those on disability, it will put a huge kink in your freedom to do something new and interesting. It will also wreak havoc with your natural creativity.

Two other negative factors also work on people who manage to get a diagnosis of permanent disability. One is low-level fear based on the worry that if they heal up, they will have to go back to doing what they did before. If this was something they disliked, they have very little incentive to get well again.

The other negative factor is low-level guilt that they have succeeded in getting out of going to work. The burden of contributing to life has been put onto others. This half-unconscious guilt interferes with their freedom to do what they want to do each day. It prevents them from creating the life they might love to have because they must maintain the pretense of not being well. If they really *are* sick and disabled, the guilt is compounded with true anger, frustration, or sorrow that they cannot participate fully in what so many others do naturally and easily, and they cannot simply choose a different way of living.

The truth is that it is normal and natural to do what you want each day. It is not normal and natural to feel trapped by a corporate clock or an unnatural schedule. Neither is it normal or natural to do the same thing day after day for years on end or to do work that is not what you love to do. If your dream is to become the CEO of a large organization, then pursue it. If your dream is to study art in Italy, become a surgeon, spend your days scuba diving among sunken ruins, or become a lawyer – begin it. There is life in every decision that takes you in the direction of your dream.

Many people put off embarking on a healing program because they think they cannot take time off from work. When they are finally forced to do some serious healing, they discover that the world does not fall down if they do not show up at their office or their job. Sometimes this discovery is followed by a period of wild rebellion and a refusal to go to work at all. There is a deep recognition that the work schedule is a constant interference in life routines that would bring about full healing. This is a healthy, truthful, and often temporary rebellion, especially if one's priorities include being healthy enough to stay alive and enjoy the life you want. Without exception, when people return to true health, there is an honest and excited desire to return to the true work that sustains them. If they are no longer interested in their former work, they have the clarity, energy, and creativity to create new work, jobs, or life situations for themselves. This is true healing, through and through!

Suggestions for Creating Healing Programs

In the sample healing programs that follow, I hope you will see that all of the pieces that support good health are put together in a variety of creative and useful ways that bring the body back to health and balance. The art of healing is truly an art. Each person and the problems they present form a set of conditions. The true healer looks at all of those conditions and uses every tool at his or her disposal to bring the body back to health. All of the pieces presented earlier in this book are your tools. Use whatever tool you need to get the job done. Learning how to use the natural tools that are available to us all will give you a feeling of security and confidence in terms of taking care of yourself and your family. This is sustainable medicine at its best.

In the sample healing programs listed here, you will find suggestions on how to use the major tools of food, supplements, exercise, and detox, as well as other useful substances like herbs or practices such as packs or soaks. You might not use all of the suggestions in every case, but I list them because they are so powerful when used together.

❖

Diarrhea

Diarrhea is very common and can accompany illnesses like the flu, irritable bowel syndrome, food poisoning, food allergies, taking too many laxatives, cancers, the result of chemotherapy and radiation, parasites, and many other conditions. The following are things that I would do. The first two help almost immediately.

Clay – Bentonite clay not only stops diarrhea, it heals the intestinal tract, soaks up poisons, kills parasites, and does an amazing job overall. Keep it on hand in powder form and mix 1 tsp in a half-glass of warm water and drink 1-3 times a day. You can also buy Sonne's or Progressive Labs' Bentonite Clay in liquid suspension and take 1 TBSP 1-3 times a day until the diarrhea subsides.

Charcoal – If the diarrhea is severe, I would take 4 capsules of charcoal every hour until it stops, using only a small amount of water and *not* taking anything else by mouth, including food, medicine, or supplements. Charcoal tablets can be purchased at your local health food store. When the diarrhea has stopped and your gastrointestinal system is quiet, leave it that way for 24 hours, taking small sips of water frequently, but not eating anything.

Then begin the following, eating tiny amounts – a mouthful at a time – for the first day or two.

Foods that help prevent the return of the diarrhea would be:

- Ripe bananas in small doses
- Peanutbutter (real, freshly ground is preferred, from a spoon, not on toast)
- One or two ounces of very well-chewed beef. Chew small pieces 30-40 times each
- Mashed potatoes, not too much seasoning, just a dash of salt, no pepper, no butter or margarine
- Oatmeal or brown rice in small doses, 1-2 TBSP at a time

- Foods to avoid would be beans of any kind, caffeine, fruit, (especially unripe fruit), any packaged or processed foods.

Digestive enzymes

- Once the diarrhea is past and I could eat without triggering it again, I would begin taking 1 Super Digestaway capsule (by Solaray) with each meal to help with stomach digestion, and 2 Pancreas enzyme capsules to help with intestinal digestion and absorption of nutrients.

Supplements *(15 days on/5 days off)*

- 2 capsules Acidophilus on an empty stomach, 2 x day, before breakfast and at bedtime

- Vitamin C, 1000 mg, 4-6 x day

- Vitamin B-Complex 100s, 3 x day

- A calcium-magnesium supplement with a ratio of 500 mg calcium/250 mg magnesium, 2 x day, at breakfast and bedtime

- 2 TBSP flaxseed oil *every* day! Put it on a salad with your regular dressing over it to cover the taste; or in oatmeal; in warm – not hot – soup; or on mashed potatoes, steamed veggies, etc.

- ½ cup yogurt, 3 x day

- Glutathione, 500 mg, 2 x day, an anti-oxidant to help deal with the by-products created by the relatively poor digestion and other conditions in the body

- Coenzyme Q-10, 100 mg/day

- A good multi-vitamin/mineral capsule, 2 x day. It should have at least 8,000-10,000 iu of Vitamin A and some amount of calcium and magnesium in correct ratio of 2 mg calcium to 1 mg magnesium. (Do not reduce the calcium-magnesium supplement recommended above unless the total amount of calcium goes over 1,500 mg/day. You want to shoot for a total calcium intake of not more than 1,500 mg/day.)

- If you are recovering from surgery, you can take a total of 100,000 iu of Vitamin A for 5 days straight, then drop to 50,000 iu for 5 days, then drop to 25,000 iu, and maintain that for 5 days. Then do not take *any* Vitamin A for 5 days. After that, there should be sufficient healing to go on a maintenance dose of

15,000 iu per day. *No healing can take place without sufficient quantities of Vitamin A regardless of what else you are taking.* However, do NOT take huge amounts of Vitamin A for more than a month without a break of at least 5 days. When you are seriously ill, your body can use the larger doses, but when you have recovered, it can build up in the body, become toxic, and can cause the brain to swell.

- When taking ANY vitamin or supplement program, don't forget, the rule is "15 days on, 5 days off." Do not take vitamins and minerals or other supplements continuously. They cause such a furious rate of repair, replacement, and rebuilding that the body can actually bog down in its rate of healing if you don't give it a brief rest from all supplements. If you have had a serious operation or illness, get out a calendar and write on it what you need to be taking and when. Once that's done, just refer to the calendar, otherwise you'll forget, get confused, etc. It is well worth the effort to be organized in terms of your own healing programs.

Making Notes

It is a good idea to write out or type and print your healing programs, make dated notes on them of what worked, what you experienced, and, if there was a sequence of changes that you went through, what these changes were. Keep these written or typed programs and notes in a notebook or file them in a file called "Family Healing Programs" or something similar.

Quite often when you are trying to put together a healing program for yourself or a family member, something will come to you intuitively. You may not have any particular reason why you think such-and-so should be done, or avoided, or eaten, or practiced...but it keeps popping into your mind. This is often a key piece of the total healing program! Don't ignore it.

Later, if the condition returns, many people get anxious and fear they won't heal properly again because they can't recall all of the little intuitive things they did that first time to bring about healing. If it's all written down, it's right there. If there is a new intuitive flash or two, add that to the program. If something doesn't seem quite necessary from the old program, don't do it. Healing is an *art* even more than a science. The science part is in knowing what effects a particular food, mineral, or herb, etc., will have on *most* people. The art is in assembling the right pieces to support *your* body's healing work, and then adding or subtracting from the program based on your past experience, intuitions, and current observations. The body is a dynamic, living system. What is healing during one episode of illness may not necessarily work, or work as well, in the next episode. Many factors affect this – the nature of the illness, the conditions in the body, the seasons, the amount of stress going on at that period in life, things like age, sex, relationships, diet, physical activity, and the stage of the illness. Thus, your intuition is a critical part of your healing program. Use it!

Cataracts, Detached Retina, and Eye Diseases

Cataracts, macular degeneration, and retina problems can often be stopped and even reversed if you embark on a healing program specifically designed to support your eyes. Although it may seem like a lot of work, your eyes are well worth it. The following is an example of a fairly complete program.

Detox

- Drink at least 8-10 glasses of R.O. water *every* day.

- Do a Liver Flush as outlined earlier. The first day of the Liver Flush is Day 1 of your healing program.

- Two weeks from the date you started the Liver Flush begin a Colon Sweep, being careful to eat plenty of yogurt and take acidophilus afterwards.

- Two weeks from the date you started the Colon Sweep, begin a 3-day diet of fresh fruits and salad, then do the 2-day version of the Purge, followed by another 3 days of fresh fruit and salad.

Transition

- For 3 days after you finish the Purge, eat at least ½ cup of yogurt with each meal. At each bedtime, take 2 Acidophilus capsules on an empty stomach.

Supplements (15 days on/5 days off)

- Amino acids in a balanced formula, 1 capsule/day, with water, in the morning, on an empty stomach. (A balanced formula means that the capsule contains the correct amount of each amino that you generally need, and all the amounts are in the correct ratios to one another.)

- Flaxseed oil 2 TBSP/day, or Evening Primrose oil, 1000 mg, 3 x day

- Vitamin A in emulsion form, 50,000 iu/day for 5 days, then drop to 25,000 iu/day for 5 days, then drop to 15,000 iu/day for 5 days. Then stop all vitamins for 5 days. Then begin again, and thereafter take 15,000 iu/day for the rest of the program.

- Vitamin C, 3,000 mg, 4 x day, for the first two rounds of 15 days on/5 days off. Next, take 2,000 mg, 3 x day for one round of 15 days on/5 days off. Thereafter, take 1,000 mg, 3 x day as maintenance. Vitamin C prevents the rupture and resulting scars in tiny capillaries that feed the eyeball, retina, and other eye structures. If you have a history of kidney stones, be careful about taking Vitamin C in higher doses. You may want to lower the dose to 500 mg, 2-3 x day throughout the healing program.

- Beta Carotene, 25,000 iu/day

- Copper, 3 mg/day

- Manganese, 10 mg/day (Always take manganese separately from calcium.)

- Glutathione, 500 mg, 1 x day or 250 mg, 2 x day

- Selenium, 400 mcg/day

- A *balanced* Vitamin B-Complex capsule, 1 x day

- L-Lysine, 500 mg, 1 x day, taken at the same time as the Vitamin B-Complex capsule above

- Additional Vitamin B-1, 50 mg/day

- Additional Vitamin B-2, 50 mg/day

- Additional Vitamin B-5 (pantothenic acid) 500 mg, 1 x day

- Vitamin E (mixed tocopherols), 400 iu, 1 x day

- Zinc, 15 mg, 3 x day

- Bilberry, 480 mg/day

- Pycnogenol (grape seed extract), as directed on the bottle

- A multiple-vitamin/multiple-mineral supplement containing the basic vitamins and at least the 6 major minerals (calcium, magnesium, sodium, potassium, iron, and zinc) described in the chapter on *Supplements*, 2 x day

Exercise is absolutely necessary when healing eyes.

- Every morning when you wake up and before you get out of bed, squeeze your eyes shut tightly, then open them as widely as possible, alternating these two eye movements 10 times. Then rotate your eyeballs in a circle, looking as far *up* as possible, then to the *left*, then *down* as far as possible, then to the *right* as far as possible, and back up. Rotate 25 times in one direction, then reverse and rotate 25 times in the opposite direction. Then close your eyes and relax them for a few minutes before getting out of bed.

- Sit facing the sun, with eyes closed, and very slowly move your head back and forth from left to right, for 15-20 minutes each day, allowing the sun to hit the closed eyes.

- Walk briskly for 10-15 minutes on two successive days, then skip a day, and walk again for two additional days. Then skip two days. Walk two days, skip 1, walk 2, skip 2. Repeat throughout the program.

- *After you have been taking the Vitamin C* for the first two rotations of 15 days on/5 days off and are past the danger of rupture in small blood vessels and capillaries at the back of the eye, take up the following...

- Do 10-15 minutes of stretching in the late afternoon, ending by bending forward from the waist, letting your arms dangle toward the floor (or resting on the floor if you're more flexible) and letting the blood flow into the head. Work at breathing as normally as possible while bent over, for at least 5 minutes, less when you first try this, longer as you get used to it. If you have high blood pressure, for the first two weeks lean forward from the waist, clasping your elbows, and resting both head and arms on a table, or a chair, letting blood flow toward your head and breathing deeply, exhaling completely.

Food & Sleep

Eat whole, natural foods as much as you can. Avoid sweets like the plague. Getting a bit of extra sleep is critical during the first three months of healing your eyes, so say goodnight to everyone a couple hours earlier than usual and retire to your room. Even if you don't go to bed immediately, this should help lower stress and make it easier for you to go to bed at least one hour early. If you don't go to sleep right away, that's okay, too. Just lay there with your eyes closed and breathe deeply, as if breathing living light energy into your eyeballs. You can also daydream, think, plan, envision, or do a few more eye exercises. All of these are very healing for your eyes.

You do not need to give up coffee or tea completely while healing your eyes, but it is good to cut back for a while because caffeine draws water out of your tissues, leaving them dry and unable to function properly. Also, avoid drinking a cup of coffee after you have just eaten. Not only does the caffeine interfere with the absorption of nutrients, most people want a cup of coffee after meals for two reasons, neither of them conscious.

The first reason is that they ate too much and instinctively want to hurry that full feeling away by stimulating their body to move the meal quickly onward through their gastrointestinal system. However, hurrying things along will mean that the food is only partially digested, and you will not get the full benefit of the nutrients in it. This is a waste of your food dollar and a burden on the body instead of an asset.

The other reason is that when you eat, your adrenals and pancreas must go into overdrive to digest the food. For many people, the adrenals and pancreas are near exhaustion from too much stress and pressure, too much food, and too little nutrition and rest. Digestion, which is a huge burden on the body, takes so much effort that when the adrenals and pancreas are exhausted, people feel tired, sleepy, fatigued, and can drop into a sleepwalking state if they don't have a cup of coffee to push themselves to keep going for a few more hours. If this describes you, skip the coffee after meals and go sleep for an hour. You need it to help heal yourself and allow time for the best digestion.

❖

Prostate Troubles & Urinary Difficulties (Men)

Supplements (15 days on/5 days off)

- Amino acids in a balanced formula, 1 capsule/day, with water, in the morning, on an empty stomach. (A balanced formula means that the capsule contains the correct amount of each amino that you generally need, and all the amounts are in the correct ratios to one another.)

- Flaxseed oil, 2 TBSP/day, on salads, in warm soups, or over steamed vegetables with butter (to cover the taste) *or* Evening Primrose oil capsules, at least 350 mg, 6 x day, taking 2 at breakfast, 2 at lunch, and 2 at dinner

- Zinc in picolinate form, 60 mg/day for 3 months, then reduce to 45 mg/day for 3 months, then reduce to 30 mg/day for maintenance

- Vitamin C, 1,000 mg, 4 x day

- A *balanced* Vitamin B-Complex capsule, 3 x day

- Vitamin E, 400 iu, 2 x day

- Additional Vitamin B-6, 100-250 mg, 1 x day

- Copper, 2 mg, 1 x day

- Saw palmetto berry capsules, 160 mg, 2 x day

- Vitamin A, 15,000 iu, 1 x day

Food & Water

- Drink 64 oz of water every day, no days off, no excuses.

- For a time, *limit* alcohol, stress, and coffee until the symptoms recede and healing has a good start.

- Limit commercial chicken for 3-4 months because it is often loaded with estrogens, which play a role in the swelling of the prostate.

- Make and drink 1 pint of carrot juice, 3 x week.

- Take 3 digestive enzymes with each meal: 1 Super Digestaway capsule (by Solaray) and 2 Pancreas Glandular enzymes.

- Alternate daily: ½ cup of pumpkin seeds on Day 1; ½ cup of sunflower seeds on Day 2; 10 almonds on Day 3, then begin again.

Exercises

- Walk briskly for 30-60 minutes each day for two days, skip one day, then walk briskly for two more days, then skip two days. Then begin again. The walking not only increases circulation to the affected areas, it raises your level of energy, which is important for the male ego.

- On the days that you are not walking, lie down on the floor next to a wall, with your body perpendicular to the wall. Raise your legs straight up and rest them against the wall. Lie there with your legs up the wall for at least 10 minutes, less in the beginning if necessary, and more if you can, as you build yourself toward good health.

- Do a set of 25 Kegle exercises every morning and every night. These are simple. Just stand in place and tighten up all of the muscles you would normally use to stop urination, count to 3, then relax. This tightens the lower abdomen, upper legs, hips, and works all of the organs in the lower part of the body.

- Do not avoid lovemaking altogether, but don't engage in prolonged lovemaking. If you do not have a spouse or lover, yet still have a functioning sex drive, masturbate through to ejaculation routinely to keep things moving in the genital area. Saw palmetto berry tends to accentuate your sexuality, so don't fight your own healing or wonder what has gotten into you lately that you're suddenly in need of more sexual activity.

- Do a Salt and Soda Bath twice each week for 6 weeks.

Notes

You should notice significant improvement in 4-6 weeks on this healing program, but should stay on it for at least 3 months and go a full 6 months if you can.

Once your prostate and urinary habits have returned to normal, you can go off the saw palmetto and embark on a full detox program and a regular supplement program, with careful attention to diet and ongoing stretching and walking. If the prostate difficulties return, which is unlikely if you're still taking the full spectrum of vitamin and mineral supplements, keeping up with your exercise, and including the flaxseed oil, then start taking the saw palmetto again for another 3-6 months while continuing to reduce stress and improve your lifestyle.

Depression

If you are seriously depressed, all of the diet, exercise and supplement changes recommended throughout this book should help tremendously.

If you are too depressed to put together a healing program and get yourself started with it, then consider taking a specific form of amino acid called *S-adenosyl L-methionine E*, aka SAM-e, (pronounced săm-ē′). This is a form of methionine that supports your mitochondria in their efforts to produce the adenosine triphosphate (ATP) that gives you the energy you need for living and enjoying life.

SAM-e must be taken with Vitamin B-6, Vitamin B-12, and Folic acid or it won't work, but many SAM-e tablets include these vitamins right in the tablet. If they are not included in the tablets you buy, then get some B-Complex 25 (or B-Complex 50) from your local health food store and take 1 capsule twice a day.

The usual way to take SAM-e is to start with what is known as a *loading dose* at first, then drop gradually until you get to the maintenance dose. For many people, this is:

1,000 mg/day, divided into 2-4 doses, for two weeks, then drop to

800 mg/day, in divided doses, for two weeks, then drop to

600 mg/day, in divided doses, for two weeks, then drop to

400 mg/day, in divided doses, for two weeks, then drop to

200 mg/day, in divided doses, and stay there for 3 months.

At the end of the 3 months at the 200 mg/day level, you might try dropping to 100 mg/day and see if you maintain your good energy and steady spirits. If not, go back up to the 200 mg/day and stay there for another 3 months. Do not take SAM-e for more than 6 months without a break. It is a wonderful supplement, and research has not been able to come up with any side effects, but you don't want to tempt fate. Take a 2-3 week break from it and rely on good nutrition to keep you out of the pits.

Detox is critical in eliminating depression.

- While you are off the SAM-e, **do a Liver Flush**. When the liver is congested, depression is almost guaranteed. At the very least, you will be irritable, blue, and lethargic. Sometimes doing a *Liver Flush* is all that is needed to lift depression entirely.

- Two weeks later **do a Colon Sweep**. This will help the assimilation of nutrients into your system, which helps with your energy.

- Two weeks later **do the Purge** to remove wastes throughout your body.

- Continue doing this rotation of three detox procedures, one each month for the next year.

- Commit to doing a set of Coffee Enemas every evening to keep the liver clear, since a sluggish or plugged liver is a major factor in depression.

- When you are finished with the first round of detox procedures, return to taking a maintenance-level dose of SAM-e. (You do not need to repeat the loading dose unless you've been off SAM-e for more than three months.)

Food

- In between detox procedures, begin changing your diet to the best, whole, high-nutrition food you can get your hands on. Commit to a basic diet and exercise program that will be good for you and keep your spirits up. Eat the entire spectrum of foods: meat, fish, eggs, cheese, butter, milk, whole grains, plenty of vegetables, and fresh fruits, avoiding only those things you know you're allergic to.

- Do NOT eat anything with sugar in it or you're likely to end up depressed again. Eliminate sugar, processed foods, and foods with little or no nutrition. These lead to serious depression over time, which is why half of our nation is suffering from depression. Learn to shop differently. Learn to prepare meals differently.

- Eat 3-4 small meals each day, rather than one or two snacks and then a huge meal all at once. Eat quietly, and chew thoroughly.

Exercise often eliminates depression!

- Be sure to exercise because this forces the delivery of nutrients into the far corners of the body as well as through any resistant cell membranes. *The Fountain Of Youth Exercises* are particularly helpful here because they work on the endocrine system so effectively, which is implicated in depression. Walking, swimming, running, biking, dancing, and even gardening are very helpful in relieving depression.

Supplements

- Amino acids in a balanced formula, 2 capsules/day, with water, one in the morning and one at bedtime, on an empty stomach. (A balanced formula means that the capsule contains the correct amount of each amino that you generally need, and all the amounts are in the correct ratios to one another.)
- Vitamin B-Complex 100, 2 capsules/day
- Vitamin C, 1000 mg, 2 x day
- Take a good, multiple vitamin/multiple mineral capsule from a reputable manufacturer, 2 x day, with meals.
- Flaxseed oil, 2 TBSP/day, on salad, in soup, in smoothies, or straight from the spoon
- Adrenal glandular, as directed on the bottle
- Digestive enzymes (SuperDigestaway), 1 with each meal
- Pancreas glandular supplement, 2 with each meal

Notes

For many people, depression is the result of malnutrition and exhaustion. Exhaustion can be caused by stress, poor relationships, and many other factors. Evaluate your job, your relationships, and your goals in life. Begin to live the life you are interested in. Don't ever shortchange yourself because you think you owe something to someone else! There is no situation that cannot be handled well if you put a little mature thinking and compassion into how to do so. The stress of trying to lie to yourself or deny yourself, drains the body and leaves it unable to produce the neurochemicals that allow you to maintain comfortable emotional and mental states. Poor nutrition, an over-loaded colon, and a poorly working liver then complicate this biochemical imbalance. The result is depression.

With the restoration of a steady supply of ATP, clearing the liver and colon, high-density nutrition, and a bit of exercise, the results can be magical in a really short time. As you slowly rebuild your body/mind system, you'll find you can maintain good energy and a sense of well-being without the SAM-e. Although SAM-e is not bad for you, it is on the pricey side, although much cheaper than prescriptions. And it's even cheaper still to get the same effect from good food and a lifestyle that supports good health.

Infections – Bacterial, Viral, or Fungal

Detox

- Drink 8 oz of water every hour to equal 1 gallon of water daily.

- *Stop eating.* If you have a serious bacterial infection, do not eat at all. Do a complete water fast for 4-10 days, drinking one 8 oz glass of water every hour each day until you have consumed one gallon.

- As soon as you realize you have an infection, mix together the following trace mineral "cocktail":

- ¼ tsp of liquid trace minerals by ConcenTrace (to help kill the infection). Quantities of trace minerals will cause loose bowels and diarrhea.

- ½ cup of orange juice, to cover the taste of the trace minerals

- ½-1 TBSP of Bentonite clay in suspension, by Sonné, to prevent diarrhea. The bowels may be loose, and you will get cleaned out, but you don't want uncontrolled diarrhea.

Every 2 hours for the first 8 hours, make one of these trace mineral cocktails and drink immediately. For the next five days, make and drink one trace mineral cocktail 4 x day until infection is gone. Drink the mineral cocktail in between the 8 oz glasses of water. Trace minerals are very powerful; I have seen nasty post-surgical infections clear up within 3-5 days using trace minerals.

Alternate plan, in case you don't have the trace minerals and Bentonite clay on hand and can't get them quickly:

- 1 tsp of colloidal silver in a cup of water 2 x day. Silver is not as powerful as the trace minerals, but it does an excellent job. Be sure to stop taking the colloidal silver after 10 days because it is known to cause patches of gray, discolored skin that do not return to their natural color. If the gray patch were to appear on your face, you would be quite unhappy about it.

- 500 mg of garlic, 3 x day until the infection has cleared up

Food

- When you do begin eating again, *no* alcohol, sugar, or caffeine! These make the body too acid, which is the perfect environment for *bacterial* infections. Sugar feeds infections, while alcohol and caffeine draw water out of your tissues, something you cannot afford during an infection. Instead, stick to fresh raw citrus fruits, fresh raw vegetable juices, and beef broth or chicken broth. An alkaline environment is preferred by viruses and fungi, therefore avoid citrus juice if you have a viral infection since citrus alkalinizes the body. Drink milk instead, which acidifies the body.

- Carrot/Garlic Juice – make 1 pint of carrot juice every day (about 6-10 carrots, depending on size). Juice 1 large clove of garlic into the juice. Drink immediately.

- Lemon/honey/cayenne drink – Mix 2 TBSP of fresh lemon juice, 1 TBSP honey, 1/8 tsp of cayenne, and 2 cups of water in a quart pan. Heat until warm, but do not boil. Drink 1 cup in the morning and 1 cup in the afternoon. Do not warm in the microwave. In fact, do not use a microwave for anything.

- Put 1 teabag of Red Clover and 1 teabag of Burdock Root into a teapot and cover with 2 cups of boiling water. Steep 15 minutes, then drink 1 cup mid-morning and 1 cup mid-afternoon each day to help clean the blood. Continue this for three months.

Healing Procedures

- Clay pack (green clay if possible), 1 inch thick, directly over the infected area for at least 2 hours each day, unless the infection is in an incision. In that case, put the clay on an adjacent section of the body, at least four or five inches away.

- Do a Castor Oil Pack on the abdomen to stimulate the immune system, 2 hours each day for 5 days, then take 3 days off, use the pack again for 5 days, then 3 days off, and continue to rotate until the infection is cleared up. Do not use the Castor Oil Pack directly over an incision until it is completely healed as the pack is not sterile enough. If you have an incision in your abdomen, place the pack on your chest.

- If you don't have a Castor Oil Pack, use a heating pad to heat the area for two hours, as bacteria do not have much tolerance for temperatures over 106°. My husband spent a week in the hospital with a terrible leg infection and all kinds of intravenous antibiotics, but it was a heating pad that finally turned the tide toward healing.

- On the 3 days off from the Castor Oil Pack, use alternating hot and cold packs, 15-20 minutes for the hot pack and about 5 minutes for the cold pack. Keep alternating for 1 hour.

- If the infection is in a hand or foot, soak the affected area in a large pan of hot water, 1 cup of Epsom Salt, and 1 cup of ordinary salt (sodium chloride) twice a day.

- If the infection is in an arm or leg, soak your entire self in a Salt and Soda Bath.

- Soak a fungal infection by rubbing the infected area with tea tree oil, soaking in hot water for 20-30 minutes, drying the affected part, then coating with tea tree oil again.

- If the infection is athlete's foot, put 2 TBSP of colloidal silver in a basin of warm water and soak your feet for 20-30 minutes, twice a day.

Supplements (15 days on/5 days off) until the infection is healed...

- A good vitamin/mineral capsule, 3 x day
- Vitamin C, 1,000 mg, 4-6 x day
- Vitamin A, 25,000 iu, 3 x day
- Zinc, 15 mg, 4 x daily
- Vitamin E, 400 iu, 1 x day
- Co-enzyme Q-10, 100 mg, 3 x day

- Hydrogen Peroxide, 3% strength, 1 tsp in 1 cup of water, and drink daily

- Bromelain capsules, 500 mg, 3 x day, with the lemon/honey/cayenne drink if possible

- Avoid taking iron when you have a bacterial infection, as bacteria tend to use the iron for their own strength and benefit

- When the infection is gone, continue to take the above supplements for another two weeks. Then switch to a good amino acid capsule and multiple vitamin/multiple mineral supplement on a daily basis. Continue drinking at least 8-10 glasses of water each day.

Exercise

- If possible, stretch, dance, or walk briskly for 15-30 minutes each day.

- Light massage all around the infected area is very helpful and speeds healing tremendously.

- Rest, rest, and rest some more.

Cancers and AIDS

Detox

- Do the Liver Flush as described earlier in the book. The first day of the Liver Flush is Day 1 of your healing program.

- Two weeks from Day One, begin the Colon Sweep.

- Four weeks from Day One, do The Purge, making and drinking the citrus punch for three days instead of two.

- Immediately after completing these three detox procedures, begin doing at least two sets of Coffee Enemas each day, one set in the morning and another set in the evening. If you are doing chemo or radiation, the number of Coffee Enemas can go up as the amount of dead cancer tissue circulating in your body goes up. Remember, the liver is responsible for keeping these poisons out of circulation, and because dead tumor tissue is so incredibly toxic, the liver can be quickly overwhelmed, causing you to feel nauseous, full of aches, pain, fatigue and fear. The Coffee Enema is an important and powerful tool for keeping the liver functioning and your spirits up.

Food & Water

- **Drink reverse osmosis water, a minimum of 64 oz per day**, preferably 128 oz. Do *not* drink tap water, especially if it has been chlorinated to kill germs or fluoridated to "prevent cavities." Drinking ½ to 1 gallon of water a day is non-negotiable if you want to heal cancer.

- Carrot/Garlic Juice – twice a day make 1 pint of carrot juice. Juice 1 large clove of garlic into the juice and drink immediately. You can add a couple stalks of celery, an apple, a slice or two of beet, or other vegetable for variety.

- If you are going to have surgery, *stop taking garlic at least 3 weeks beforehand.* Garlic makes the blood very fluid and reduces clotting. You do not want your doctor to end up with a case of uncontrolled bleeding during your surgery.

- Switch to organic foods as much as possible in order to reduce the amount of heavy metals and poisonous chemicals you take in. Many of these metals and chemicals seriously derange your endocrine system, and only a few molecules of a heavy metal are needed to create this havoc.

- As much as possible, do not drink anything with caffeine or alcohol in it during the healing process.

- Do not eat anything with white flour or white sugar in it, no boxed cereals, and *no* soy products. The white flour products and pastas, boxed cereals, and sugar have little or no usable nutrition in them. Sugar supports the growth of tumors and also shuts down your immune system for up to four hours, something you cannot really afford when you are healing cancer or AIDS. White flour products, cereals, and soy all prevent absorption of much-needed minerals that help repair and rebuild the body. According to Dr. Gonzales and research from the Price-Pottenger Foundation, soy products disrupt the endocrine system. They also destroy crucial enzymes that your body produces to fight cancer, and they substitute their own enzymes that do not work as well, if at all. Make or buy breads and rolls with freshly ground, whole wheat flour in them, and choose old-fashioned pastas made with whole wheat, butter, and eggs.

- Make 14-Grain Cereal and eat it 3-4 times a week. Use organic grape juice or apple juice to soak the grain overnight.

- Make a very good beef broth regularly and either sip the broth as a drink or make homemade soup with it.

- Every day eat a very large salad made from 30% dark greens and the rest chopped, raw vegetables. Put your flaxseed or hempseed oil on it, then put your regular salad dressing on top of that to cover the taste.

- Eat 10 raw almonds every day to help alkalinize the body if you are too acid. Eat 10 raw walnuts every day to help acidify the body if you are too alkaline.

- Have your blood tested for its pH balance (its acid/alkaline balance). If you are too acid (below 6.6 pH), begin changing your diet to eat large amounts of raw vegetables and fruits, and drink a cup of hot water with the juice of one lemon in it once or twice a day. If you are too alkaline, (above 7.4 pH) change your diet to include red meat, cheese, and dairy products every day until your system is back in balance. Have your acid/alkaline balance tested every three months to see where you are at so you can eat accordingly.

To determine whether you are too acid or too alkaline, get a *comprehensive* blood test, sometimes called a *full chemical scan* or a *CMP*, and ask for a copy of the test results. You can also arrange for a hair test, and this test often tells you which heavy metals are in your system as well as how much of them you have ingested.

When doctors do what they call "a full blood work-up," the report includes your blood pH. Ask for a copy of the report so you will know which way you are leaning – too acid or too alkaline. If you don't have a recent blood test and don't want to get one, get some pH paper from your local pharmacist. They can usually order it for you if they don't have it on hand. Although this is not nearly as reliable as a blood test, it will at least give you an idea of where you are leaning. Put the pH paper, which comes in a roll like scotch tape, in your bathroom and every morning for one week test the pH of your urine in the following way.

Get up in the morning and without eating or drinking anything, go directly to the bathroom. Tear about 2-4 inches of pH paper from the roll. Sit on the toilet and begin to go to the bathroom. Before you finish urinating, about midway through the process, stick the pH paper in the stream of urine and then withdraw it. Quickly compare it to the color charts on the pH paper dispenser. I say "quickly" because it will begin to dry quickly and change color. Keep a record of the dates, times, and readings of each pH test.

The normal condition of first morning urine should be somewhat acid, maybe between 6.0 and 6.5 pH. If yours is down below the 6.0 pH range, you are leaning toward the acid side. If it is up in the 7.5 range or above, you are too alkaline.

About three hours later, after you've eaten and drank, test your pH again and compare this with the early morning test results. It should be a little less acid, perhaps around 6.6 or 6.7 pH. If you are even more acid, this confirms that you are too acid. If the pH paper shows that you are still way up in the alkaline range, then it's time to begin adjusting your diet.

Test yourself at least twice more over the course of the day for about five days, always recording the date, time, and pH reading. You should notice that your pH is lower when you get up in the morning and goes up over the course of the day, depending on what you eat. What you want is to determine where you are most of the time.

If you are too acid, your cell membranes will close up tightly and nothing will be able to get in or out of your cells. Even if you are eating the best foods possible and taking supplements, you will not be getting the benefit of this good nutrition because the cells cannot open up enough to allow the available nutrients in. Acid conditions in the body create *sclerosis,* or hardening of tissues, and being too acid is a slow route to malnutrition and degeneration.

If you are too alkaline, the cell membranes will be too loose and open. Not only will the hundreds of toxins in our world get into the cell interior to do serious damage to mitochondria and other internal cellular structures, they will derange cellular function. Your efforts to supply the cell with needed nutrients for repair and rebuilding will be thwarted because the nutrients will flow in and flow right out again due to the extreme permeability of the cell wall. Overly alkaline conditions in the body not only cause a too-drastic softening of tissues to the point they begin to break down, but this opens you to attack by every virus and toxin that's out there.

Correcting your pH is necessary for healing, balance within the body, and support of your immune system. It is also critical for optimal absorption, retention, and use of minerals and vitamins. Using pH paper is not an optimal method for determining your acid-alkaline balance, but it will give you an idea of which way to go with your diet. It can take some time to change your pH permanently; often at least six months, and sometimes a year or two is necessary to shift the acid/alkaline balance and stabilize it at the new position.

When you are too acid, you need to eat a diet based heavily in salads and vegetables, especially raw ones. When you're too alkaline you need to eat a diet based heavily in proteins from meat and dairy. Blood pH should be somewhere between 6.9 and 7.2. Rarely is it 7.0 because this is neutral and not helpful in terms of chemical reactions! If you're 7.1 or 7.2, you're in a reasonable state. If you're more than 5 points above or below the ideal, you should start making changes in diet.

Some people use the pH paper to test their saliva, but the pH of your saliva is much more unstable. Just breathing through your mouth will change the pH of saliva, making it more acid, which is why people who breathe through their mouth have more cavities than those who breathe through their nose. I recommend the urine test, or better yet, a blood test to get a more accurate picture of what you need to do.

Supplements (15 days on/5 days off)

- Amino acid capsule with 23-29 L-form aminos in it, 2 x day, one in the morning on an empty stomach, one at bedtime on an empty stomach

- Take pancreas glandular enzymes, 425-500 mg each, 4 per meal and 4 at bedtime, with your amino acid capsule. Pancreas glandular enzymes dissolve cancerous growths and tumor tissue. *Be certain that your pancreas enzymes contain trypsin and chymotrypsin because these proteolytic enzymes are the ones that actually do the work of dissolving cancers and tumors.* Once you begin taking these enzymes, it is essential for you to do the Coffee Enemas every day and rotate through the Liver Flush, Colon Sweep, and Purge, doing one each month in a continuously rotating order because these support the liver and other tissues by removing dead cancer tissue from the body.

- As mentioned earlier, Dr. William Kelley also recommends getting up in the night at 2:30 am to take up to 12 pancreas glandular enzymes because the pancreas is quite active at that time of the day, and the intent is to support its work as fully as possible. He encourages doing this for two weeks, but also notes that if you do, you can feel quite sick, nauseous, and have symptoms that indicate the pancreas enzymes are breaking up tumors and your liver is working overtime to remove toxic waste from your body. The same thing happens during chemotherapy, and detox is invaluable at this time as well. If you are focused on breaking down old tumor material, do an additional set of Coffee Enemas, or up to six sets on the days you are feeling awful.

- In addition to pancreas enzymes, begin taking *digestive* enzyme capsules, the kind that work mainly in the stomach, 1 capsule per meal. These capsules contain things such as amylase, lipase, protease, cellulase, beet root, pancreatin, papain, bromelain, betaine HCL, ox bile extract, and herbs such as peppermint, ginger root, papaya, or aloe vera. If you buy enzymes that contain only amylase, lipase, protease, and cellulase, then consider buying a second formula that has betaine HCL and perhaps ox bile extract in it. Take 1 capsule of both with every meal.

- Flaxseed oil (an essential fatty acid or EFA), 2,000-3,000 mg/day in capsule form, or 2 TBSP of the oil every day on a salad with your regular dressing over it. You can also put it in *warm* – not hot – soup, mashed potatoes, in yogurt, or on steamed vegetables with a little butter to cover the taste. Flaxseed oil is mostly Omega 3 EFA (*alpha linolenic acid*) and does not have the required ratio of Omega 6 factors. If you take flaxseed oil, take Omega 6 capsules (*linoleic acid*), 6,000-9,000 mg/day, to keep the correct balance of EFAs. There are also flaxseed oil formulas out there now that have a nice balance of Omega 3, 6, *and* 9, although they cost more. The correct balance is: 1 pt Omega 3 to 3 pts Omega 6. Or, if you can get it, take hempseed oil. Hempseed oil contains both Omega 3 and 6 in the correct balance. The dose is the same, 2 TBSP/day on salads, in soups, or with steamed vegetables & butter. Don't hesitate to double your intake of Hempseed oil, as studies show that these essential fatty acids do an excellent job of destroying cancer. [101]

- Hydrogen Peroxide, 3% solution, 1 tsp in a cup of water, twice a day, for its oxygen

- Germanium, 3,000 mcg/day, in the morning for oxygenation.

---

[101] Erasmus, p. 272.

- DMG (dimethylglycine), as directed on the bottle, to enhance the body's ability to use available oxygen

- SOD (superoxide dismutase), as directed on the bottle, to increase the body's ability to transport oxygen

- Selenium, 200 mcg, 1 x day, in the morning so it does not interfere with sleep

- Vitamin A, 25,000 iu, 4 x day for two rounds of 15 days on/5 days off. When you start the third and fourth round of vitamins, reduce Vitamin A to 20,000 iu, 4 x day. In the fifth and sixth round, drop to 15,000 iu, 4 x day. Then drop to 10,000 iu, 4 x day for two round and maintain this amount, 15 days on and 5 days off, until healing is complete.

- A *balanced* Vitamin B-Complex capsule, 3 x day

- Vitamin C, 1,500 mg, 4 x day

- Vitamin D, 400 iu, 3 x day

- Vitamin E, 400 iu, 2-3 x day

- Co-enzyme Q-10, 100 mg, 1 x day, for its specific anti-oxidant properties and to enhance the activity of Vitamins C and E

- Glutathione, 500-1,000 mg daily, for its anti-oxidant capabilities

- Beta-carotene, 25,000 iu, 4 x daily, to allow your body to make more Vitamin A if it needs it

- If you have an estrogen-based cancer, take no more than 750 mg of calcium each day because an excess of calcium acts like the hormone estrogen and has estrogenic effects, which can complicate and worsen your condition. In addition, calcium acidifies the body and estrogens work best in an overly-acid environment. Therefore, you want to limit calcium, but you need at least some of this mineral to activate other enzymes in the body. It works best to take a small amount and take extra magnesium. The magnesium will alkalinize you and help you optimize the small amount of calcium you are taking. When dealing with an estrogen-based cancer, a good rule of thumb is to reverse the ratio and take 2 magnesium to 1 calcium. The suggested ratio, if you are too acid is 750 mg calcium to 1,500 mg magnesium. If you have an alkaline-based cancer, take 1500 mg of calcium and 750 mg. of magnesium daily.

- Potassium, 100 mg, 1 x day

- Zinc, 15 mg, 3 x day

- Iron, 18 mg, 1 x day

- Copper, 2 mg, 1 x day

- Trace Minerals, by ConcenTrace, ⅛ tsp, 2-3 x day, in juice

- Kelp, 1,000 mg/day, to support thyroid function, prevent uptake of more estrogen in the body, and provide protection against radiation

- Thymus glandular, 2 capsules/day, to support immune function

- Spleen glandular, 2 capsules/day, to support the making of red blood cells that carry oxygen

- Liver glandular, 2 capsules/day. If you have lung cancer, you may want to add lung landular, 2 capsules/day, to your supplement list. If you have ovarian cancer, add ovary glandular, 2 capsules/day.

- Melatonin, 3 mg/day, in the evening as an antioxidant

- Acidophilus, 2-3 capsules, at bedtime, with your aminos and pancreas enzymes.

Exercise:

- Alternate walking one day with stretching the next. Do 30 minutes of exercise daily.

- Do the 5 Rites from *The Ancient Secret of The Fountain Of Youth* daily to restore high levels of energy and renew your endocrine system.

- Get a massage every two weeks to assist lymph system drainage. Between massages, brush your skin daily to increase lymph drainage.

- Be aware that the most dangerous aspect of cancer is the fear that grips you and can even paralyze you from taking action. Fight this fear head-on. Use meditation, go for a long walk in a beautiful setting, and constantly re-affirm that you are alive, healthy, and loving. Find friends who will love and support the healing path you're on. Listen to positive, beautiful music.

- Use the Salt and Soda bath, the Castor Oil/Olive Oil Sweat Bath, the Mustard & Cayenne Foot Soak, and the Castor Oil Pack regularly if you experience fatigue, nausea, headache, or a general sense of malaise. Not only do they help detox your system so that you feel better, you have a sense of taking care of yourself.

Healing cancer takes time and energy, but once you have recovered, there is often a true feeling of power, humility, spirituality, and confidence that accompanies you wherever you go. You will have learned a lot about your body/mind system, much of it information that will be useful for your entire life.

Colds, Strep Throats, Upper Respiratory Trouble
Food

- **Stop eating immediately!** Do not eat again until the symptoms are gone, usually 3 to 7 days, depending on how long you delayed before beginning the activities that allow the body to heal itself. If you're really hungry, eat an orange or make a pint of carrot juice with garlic in it. Generally, if you eat anything cooked, you will notice that you feel worse, and healing will take longer. Once you have experienced the power of "not eating" to heal a cold or sore throat, you will not quibble over this fasting requirement.

- Drink a minimum of 64-128 oz of R.O. water (½-1 gal.) each day.

Detox

- Do a set of Coffee Enemas each evening until you are healed.

Healing Techniques

- Put ½-1 tsp salt in 8-10 oz hot water. Stir to dissolve, then gargle with the salt water, using it all, mouthful by mouthful. Do this at 7:00 am, 1:00 pm, and 7:00 pm each day until the symptoms have cleared and you feel well again.

- Each day, do a Salt and Soda Bath in hot water long enough to make you sweat profusely, usually 20 minutes or so.

- Stay in bed, sleep, and rest.

Supplements

- Colloidal silver, 1 tsp, 2 x day, until symptoms have cleared. Do not overdose on the colloidal silver! Follow the directions on the bottle carefully. The organic silver in solution is less likely to cause discoloration of skin or fingernails, which can be permanent.

- Vitamin C, 1,000 mg, 6-8 x day until the cold, sore/strep throat has cleared up. If you have a history of kidney stones, take only 1500 mg of Vitamin C in 500 mg increments, and stop after 5 days. Take 2 days off, then take 500 mg 3 x day, for another 5 days.

- Suck on zinc lozenges, 5 mg each, every 2-3 hours, to total not more than 9 lozenges and 45 mg zinc per day. If you have bipolar disorder, formerly called manic-depressive disorder, be cautious about using zinc and keep the total to no more than 15 mg per day.

- Vitamin A, 20,000 iu, 3-4 x day, for 7 days (a total of 60,000 – 80,000 iu/day). If you have not recovered yet, take two days off, then repeat.

- Vitamin B-Complex 100s, 2 x day

- Hydrogen peroxide, 3% solution, 1 tsp in 8 oz water, in the morning and again in the evening.

- If you know how to use homeopathic remedies, and have one that has worked for you previously, you might use that as well. Remember, when using homeopathic remedies, you have to match the *emotional habits and condition* of the sick person to the emotional habits and condition known to be characteristic of the remedy. Every homeopathic medicine is made from a substance that has an emotional fingerprint. Some substances cause a whiny or tearful mood, some make you restless, some create an irritable feeling, etc. If you become whiny and cry when sick, if you get crabby, or you feel driven to clean house and reorganize your space when you really don't feel good, these behaviors are part of the emotional expressions of illness and should be matched to the correct homeopathic fingerprint. Even if you don't know the specific emotional characteristics of some of the medicines, it is worthwhile to use homeopathics because they work so well and are fairly inexpensive. The label on each remedy will tell you what it is useful for and how much to take.

- The homeopathic remedy *Mercurius Vivus* helps the body heal strep throat in record time, much faster than antibiotics in most cases. I have also used *Hepar Sulphuricum* or *Kali Bichromicum* with good success in strep, sinus, and ear-nose-and-throat infections. If you want to learn to use homeopathic remedies, get the very excellent and user-friendly book *Everybody's Guide To Homeopathic Medicines* by Stephen Cummings, MD and Dana Ullman, MPH. [102]

Sinus Headaches or Sinus Infection

Nothing can make you as miserable as sinus problems. Be sure to check the section on *Infections* when dealing with sinus problems.

Food & Water

- For quick relief of sinus *headache*, drink 4 cups of clear water, one right after another. Your sinuses will begin to drain almost immediately, and you may begin sneezing. Continue drinking, 1 cup of water every hour that you are awake.

- If you have a sinus *infection*, drink 64 oz of plain water every day that you have the problem. Then drink another 24 oz of water with the juice of 2 lemons squeezed into it. Drink this total of 88 oz of water each day until your sinuses clear.

- **Stop** eating immediately! Do not eat again until the symptoms are gone, usually 3 to 7 days, depending on how long you delayed before beginning the activities that allow the body to heal itself. Sinus trouble of any kind is a clear indication you are eating foods that do not agree with your body and its needs. Constant sinus problems also indicate that you either have, or are developing, allergies.

---

[102] See Appendix B, *Suggested References,* for more information about this book.

Healing Techniques

- Do a Liver Flush. Poor diet and a plugged or sluggish liver is often a root cause of sinus problems.

- Do the 5 Rites from *The Ancient Secret of The Fountain of Youth* in the morning and the evening. These five exercises have an amazing ability to get the sinuses to drain. You can do them 3 or 4 times a day if necessary; they only take a few minutes.

- Do a set of Coffee Enemas in the morning and again in the afternoon if you feel nauseous.

- Do either the Salt and Soda Bath or the Castor Oil/Olive Oil Sweat Bath.

Supplements

- If you have a full-blown sinus infection, follow the directions for using trace minerals under *Infections* on pages 250-253.

- Colloidal silver, 1 tsp, 2 x day until the infection is gone. Again, do not overdose on the colloidal silver as it can cause skin discolorations that have a tendency to stay.

- Homeopathic remedy *Kali Bichromicum*, sometimes just called *Kali* or *Kali Bi*. Dissolve 3 tablets under your tongue once per hour for 3 hours. This is a total of 3 doses and 9 tablets. After the third dose, wait 6 hours then take 3 more tablets. This ends your first day's dose. The second day, take 3 tablets three times, with about 4 hours in between each dose. You should be feeling much better by the end of the second day, especially if you are drinking a sufficient amount of water. If the homeopathic remedy isn't working by the end of the second day, try a different remedy for two more days.

- If you have a sinus headache rather than a full-blown infection, the *Kali Bichromicum* helps because it starts the drainage that brings relief. If you have a sinus infection, take *Mercurius Vivus* for the first 3 days, then switch to *Kali Bichromcium* for 3 more days. After that you should be doing well. D*o not eat or drink anything for 15-20 minutes before or after* taking a homeopathic remedy or you will disable the medicine and distract the body's immune system from making a good response to it.

- Vitamin C, 1,000 mg, 6 x day, until the sinus headache or infection has cleared up. Limit this to 500 mg, 3 x day if you have a history of kidney stones.

- Vitamin A, 20,000 iu, 3-4 x day, for 7 days (a total 60,000-80,000 iu)

- Vitamin B-Complex 100s, 1 x day

- Hydrogen peroxide, 3% solution, 1 tsp in 8 oz water, in the morning and again in the evening

- M-S-M (methylsufonylmethane), 1,000 mg, 3 x day. This is nutritional sulfur and helps break up infections and stringy mucous.

The Flu

Supplements

- The minute you suspect you may have the flu, stop eating and go to the health food store to get the homeopathic remedy called *Oscillococcinum*. If you feel too awful, have someone pick it up for you. Inside the package, there will be 3 small vials containing tiny white beads of the remedy. Open 1 vial and pour the contents under your tongue, letting the beads dissolve. Do not eat or drink anything. Go to bed and stay there until it is time for the second dose, 6 hours later. After taking the second dose, return to bed until it is time for the third dose, 6 hours after that. This is absolutely the best flu medicine you will probably ever find. Even if you are already suffering, your flu will literally disappear within hours. If the flu hasn't quite got hold of you and you take *Oscillococcinum*, it will simply not materialize. Keep it on hand at all times.

Food

- Once you have taken the *Oscillococcinum* over the course of a day and are feeling better, eat lightly: fresh fruits, salads, beef broth with parsley in it, homemade chicken vegetable soup, steamed vegetables, whole wheat rolls or biscuits, no sweets, for a few days.

Healing Techniques

> * Take a Salt and Soda Bath for one or two nights in a row.
>
> * Do a Castor Oil Pack on your abdomen for 2-3 hrs.
>
> * Do a set of Coffee Enemas daily until recovered.

Arthritis – Rheumatoid or Osteoarthritis

If you think you have arthritis, don't hesitate a minute to begin healing because if you don't, you could end up seriously disfigured and disabled. Dr. Gonzalez once mentioned to me that at times he felt arthritis was more difficult to heal than cancer. He didn't say why he thought so, but I wondered if it was because people "fell off the wagon" (the food/detox/supplement wagon) too easily because the threat of untimely death was not part of the disease.

Water

- Drink 10-12 glasses of R.O. (reverse osmosis) water every single day, no exceptions. Water alone can erase the pain of rheumatoid arthritis within a day because most rheumatoid arthritis is triggered by chronic dehydration in the body. Without enough water, the collagen tissues in joints shrink and dry out, leaving bones and tendons to grate, become inflamed, and swell painfully.

Detox

- Do the Liver Flush to improve liver function and improve digestive processes.

- Two weeks later, do a Colon Sweep, to improve absorption of nutrients, since your joint capsules will need to be entirely rebuilt.

- Two weeks after the Colon Sweep, do the Purge to remove waste from every area of the body.

- Two weeks after the Purge, begin a series of 12 Castor Oil/ Olive Oil Sweat baths to remove wastes from the skin and allow the healing effect of castor oil to penetrate the entire body.

Food

- Begin eating whole, organic foods as much as possible. The whole food has much more nutrition in it, and eating organic will reduce the amount of heavy metals and poisonous chemicals you take in. Many of these metals and chemicals seriously derange your endocrine system, and only a few molecules of a heavy metal are needed to cause this damage.

- Get your blood tested and determine what your pH is. Stiff, sclerotic joint capsules are usually a sign of acidification. If you are too acid, begin changing your diet to a majority of fresh fruits and vegetables. Eat at least 30% raw food, which translates to at least one meal a day. Arthritis is usually the result of becoming much too acidic, however, if you are too alkaline, add red meat to your diet 3-4 x week, including beef, chicken, and fish, to bring your biochemistry into better balance.

- Carrot/Garlic Juice – twice a day make 1 pint of carrot juice. Juice 1 large clove of garlic into the juice and drink immediately. You can add a couple stalks of celery, an apple, a slice or two of beet, or other vegetable for variety.

- If you are going to have surgery to repair a joint, *stop taking garlic at least 3 weeks beforehand.* Garlic makes the blood very fluid and reduces clotting, making excess bleeding a real problem during surgery.

- As much as possible, do not drink anything with caffeine or alcohol in it during the healing process.

- Do not eat anything with white flour or white sugar in it, no boxed cereals, and *no* soy products. White flour products, cereals, and soy all prevent absorption of much-needed minerals that help repair and rebuild the joints and have little or no usable nutrition in them. According to Dr. Gonzales and research from the Price-Pottenger Foundation, soy products disrupt the endocrine system. Make or buy breads, rolls, and cereals with freshly ground, whole wheat flour in them. Choose old-fashioned pastas made with whole wheat, butter, and eggs.

- Make 14-Grain Cereal and eat it 3-4 times a week. Use organic grape juice or apple juice to soak the grain overnight.

- Make a very good beef broth regularly and either sip the broth as a drink or make homemade soup with it.

- Every day, eat a very large salad made from 30% dark greens and the rest chopped, raw vegetables. Put your flaxseed or hempseed oil on it, then put your regular salad dressing on top of that to cover the taste.

- Eat 10 raw almonds every day to help alkalinize the body if you are too acid.

Supplements (15 days on/5 days off)

- An Amino Acid capsule with at least 23-29 L-form aminos in it, 2 x day, one in the morning on an empty stomach, one at bedtime on an empty stomach

- Vitamin A, 20,000 iu, 4 x day for two rounds of 15 days on/5 days off. When you start the third round of vitamins, reduce Vitamin A to 10,000 iu, 4 x day. Maintain this amount, 15 days on and 5 days off, until healing is complete.

- Beta-carotene, 10,000 iu, 2 x daily, to allow your body to make more Vitamin A if it needs it

- A *balanced* Vitamin B-Complex capsule, 3 x day

- Vitamin C, 1,000 mg, 4 x day, unless you have a history of kidney stones, in which case you should take only 500 mg, 3 x day. Kidney stones usually form because you are much too acid, however, if you are doing the detox regularly and eating correctly, this should not be a problem.

- Vitamin D, 400 iu, 2 x day

- Vitamin E, 400 iu, 2 x day

- Co-enzyme Q-10, 30 mg, 1 x day, for its specific anti-oxidant properties and to enhance the activity of Vitamins C and E

- Calcium lactate, 750 mg, 1 x day. If you have rheumatoid arthritis, take no more than 750 mg of Calcium each day because calcium acidifies the body, which is often what you're trying to reverse in the first place. Calcium is needed to activate other enzymes in the body, but rather than take more calcium, take extra magnesium so that you will utilize all the calcium available in the body, including what you take in from food.

- Magnesium, 250-300 mg, 4 x day. The magnesium will not only help alkalinize you, it will help you optimize the small amount of calcium you are taking.

- Potassium, 100 mg, 1 x day

- Zinc, 15 mg, 2 x day

- Iron, 18 mg, 1 x day, taken between meals, on an empty stomach

- Copper, 2 mg, 1 x day

- Trace Minerals, by ConcenTrace, ¼ tsp, 1 x day, in juice

- M-S-M (methylsufonylmethane) 1,000 mg, 3 x day, for fifteen days and 5 days off. After the 5 days off, reduce to 1000 mg, 2 x day and maintain there, 1 capsule in the morning and 1 in the evening, with meals. MSM is nutritional sulfur and is used in every cell of the body to build the all-important cell membranes. M-S-M alkalinizes you and can cause diarrhea. If this occurs, reduce your dosage by one capsule each day.

Exercise

- Exercise is non-negotiable whether you have rheumatoid arthritis or osteoarthritis. Those who suffer from arthritis often stop exercising and avoid all kinds of movement because of pain or stiffness. But this is the exact opposite of what should happen. It is critically important to at least begin with some gentle stretching. Yoga is excellent for the stretching and strengthening that is needed.

- Walking is also an important form of exercise because it works the whole body. If you can add a few free weights, that is better yet, keeping in mind that the goal is to keep your core muscles in good working order.

- If you can't do anything else, start with the 5 rites in the *Fountain of Youth* exercises. [103] They not only keep you from getting worse, they restore youthfulness and energy.

- Lift free weights 3-4 times a week for a few minutes to strengthen the upper body and build muscle and tendon flexibility.

❖

---

[103] Kelder, p. 15-32.

These are only a few of the possible healing programs that are possible. When you first read through some of them, you may immediately feel overwhelmed by the number of things that are listed, and the perceived complexity of the healing processes. However, my experience has been that when you do your first Liver Flush, Coffee Enema, or Castor Oil/Olive Oil Sweat bath, you will quickly see that the reality is not nearly as overwhelming as it first appears. It is more difficult to read the list of steps that describe a process than to actually do it!

You will also find that many of the vitamins and minerals can be combined in a vitamin powder, and the exercises often turn out to be something you enjoy doing because the results are so powerful. By far, the biggest challenge is finding, trying, and getting used to new routines in the kitchen and new foods. However, once you discover the taste of real food and experience the power of natural healing, you will embrace the new lifestyle with gratitude and grace.

One day, you will look out at the world through new eyes and make comments like, "Wow, I don't know how they can eat like that!" When this happens, you will have reached a turning point in your own healing. The body is an intelligent, self-healing system. Give it what it requires and there are few illnesses and diseases that cannot be healed, or conditions that cannot be greatly improved. ❖

Part 7

Appendices

Appendix A
Personal Healing Checklist

Name _____

Condition _____

Date _____

    This section is one of the things I hand out in my classes on getting well. I created it originally for myself because I found that when I was ill, my thinking was cloudy and uncertain about what to do. I would forget the options at my fingertips. I quickly learned that the checklist was a good tool for sparking intuitions about what to do and for keeping a record of what I did to heal.

    The checklist presents the basic tools that can be used to heal yourself and serves as a reminder of the information discussed in this book. Note that the Supplements show only the Recommended Daily Allowance (RDA), which is the minimum you must take to stay alive. And remember, everyone's response to supplements is unique, so approach them as the powerful tools they are.

    In any program of healing, take into account what you put into the body and what you want to clean out. To heal permanently, you must make permanent changes in your life. Regardless of the disease or illness, recognize that *your body already knows how to heal itself.* Your job is to provide support for the body in that effort. Remember, you are the best doctor you will ever have.

Procedure	Detoxification Accomplishes	How often	Personal Need
Liver Flush	Flushes toxins, plaque, and waste materials from the liver, gall bladder, kidneys, and cardiovascular system.	Quarterly	Yes No See Chapter 16
Colon Sweep	Removes goop, yeast overgrowth, toxins, and unfriendly bacteria from the colon.	Quarterly	Yes No See Chapter 17
The Purge	Removes toxins, mucus, dead tumor tissue, dead cellular material, pus, inflamed material, and cell wastes from the entire body, but esp. lungs & joints.	Quarterly	Yes No See Chapter 18
Parasite Removal Program	Removes parasites from the tissues and G.I. tract of the body	Annual	Yes No See Chapter 24
Chelation – Intravenous EDTA	Removes plaque from the arteries.	As needed	Yes No See Chapter 21
Chelation – Subcutaneous DMPS	Removes heavy metals from the tissues of the body.	As needed	Yes No See Chapter 21
Mercury Silver Amalgams replaced with porcelain or composite	Stops the introduction of mercury into the blood & brain	Until no mercury is left in mouth	Yes No Call 1-800-331-2303 for holistic dentist in your area, or www. biocomplabs.com
Coffee enema	Causes the liver to contract, immediately dumping toxins that have accumulated there, and allows the liver to continue filtering poisons/wastes from the blood	Daily, can temporarily be needed every four hours for someone who has cancer	Yes No See Chapter 20
Fasting w. water only, Or Juice Fast	Gives the body a rest from the intense work of digestion, allows the body to catabolize poorly built cells, relieves pain, and allows rebuilding	Can be: 3-day, 5-day, 10-day, 21-day, 6-week, 3-month, or as needed	Yes No For water fast, read "Fasting Can Save Your Life" For juice fast, see "How To Get Well"

	Supplements		
Amino Acids	Provide the body with the basic materials needed to continuously rebuild its structures and tissues, fluids, enzymes, and hormones.	1 capsule daily	Yes No
Minerals	*Function*	*RDA Dose*	*Overdose*
Calcium	Supports bones and teeth; maintains regular heartbeat and transmission of nerve impulses; lowers cholesterol & risk of colon cancer; prevents muscle cramps.	800 – 1500 mg / day	Risk of kidney stones, estrogen-like effects, acidosis
Magnesium	Allows the body to utilize calcium and potassium; essential for enzyme activity; helps prevent depression and fatigue; supports lungs and heart; eases dozens of conditions from asthma to insomnia to IBS	400 – 750 mg / day	Loss of appetite, renal difficulty, diarrhea, severe edema
Sodium	Maintains proper pH, good water & fluid balance; helps prevent cramps, depression, fatigue, gas, poor memory, recurring infections, loss of taste, headache, heart palpitations, nausea, and anorexia	1100 – 3300 mg / day	Edema, high blood pressure, potassium deficiency, liver & kidney disease
Potassium	Maintains nervous system and regular heart beat; prevents stroke; lowers cholesterol; assists in transfer of nutrients through cell membranes; prevents constipation, nervousness, thirst, fatigue, headache, respiratory difficulties, and salt retention	1800 – 5600 mg / day	G.I. upset, nausea vomiting, severe fatigue, diarrhea, general weakness
Iron	Produces hemoglobin; oxygenates red blood cells; essential for enzyme activity; prevents anemia, hair loss, ridged nails, obesity, dizziness, difficulty swallowing, and slow mental reactions	18 mg / day	Constipation, digestive trouble, headache, light sensitivity, can kill under age four

Zinc	Maintains protein/enzyme synthesis; heals wounds; restores taste and smell; protects liver & prostate; assists bone formation; increases utilization of Vit. A; prevents infertility, poor memory; fights infection; speeds healing	15 mg / day	Anemia, copper deficiency, stomach upset, lethargy, impaired muscle control, lowers HDL
Vitamins	*Needed For*	*RDA Dose*	*Overdose*
Vitamin A (oil soluble)	Healing!! Maintains healthy eyes, lungs, tissues, digestive organs, bones, genitourinary tract, and cell membranes	RDA Dose: 4000-5000 iu/ day Toxic: can be as low as 25,000 iu/day in a few. Need goes up sharply when ill.	Anemia, enlarged spleen & liver, hair dry or falls out, clubbed fingers/toes, double vision, bulging fontanel
Beta Carotene (oil soluble)	Same as Vit. A, however, carotene may *not* be converted to Vit. A when diabetes, hypothyroidism, or liver malfunction is present	RDA Dose: 5000 iu / day Toxic: None	None
Vitamin B-1 Thiamine (water soluble)	Digests carbohydrates; maintains healthy appetite, digestive tract, and nervous system; protects from effects of smoking, alcohol, aging; prevents fatigue, forgetfulness, irritability	RDA Dose: 2 mg / day Toxic: 10,000 mg / day for many months	Headache, rapid pulse, trembling, weakness
Vitamin B-2 Riboflavin (water soluble)	Digests proteins, carbohydrates, and fats; maintains healthy eyes; burns calories; cracks in corners of mouth or between fingers/toes signals deficiency	RDA Dose: 1.7 mg / day Toxic: None, or very rare	Note: Riboflavin *deficiency inhibits* some cancers. Antibiotics destroy B-2
Vitamin B-3 Niacin (water soluble)	Lowers cholesterol; turns carbohydrates into energy, assists in metabolism of proteins and fats; maintains circulation and healthy skin; needed for bile and stomach fluids; reduces dementia, insomnia, low blood sugar	RDA Dose: 20 mg / day Toxic: 750 mg /day for over 3 months	Dry itchy skin, liver damage, brown pigmentation, low blood pressure, too much B-3 worsens diabetes

Vitamin B-5 Pantothenic Acid (water soluble)	Lowers stress; increases stamina; required by every cell in body; assists production of adrenal hormones, antibodies; aids metabolism; produces neurotransmitters	RDA Dose: 7 mg / day Toxic: none	None
Vitamin B-6 Pyridoxine (water soluble)	Involved in more bodily functions than any other nutrient! Maintains physical & mental health; produces enzymes & HCL; needed for DNA, RNA, & hemoglobin; metabolizes proteins, carbohydrates & fats; produces serotonin and other neurotransmitters	RDA Dose: 2 mg / day Toxic: 2000-6000 mg / day for some months	Sensory neuropathy, difficulty walking, makes allergies worse, L-dopa conflict
Vitamin B-12 Cyanocobalamin (water soluble)	Prevents anemia, helps with cell formation; required for digestion and absorption; maintains fertility; assists memory & learning; protects nerve sheaths.	RDA Dose: 3-6 Mcg./day	None, but conflicts with anti-convulsants, TB, cancer, and cholesterol drugs
Biotin (water soluble) Part of the complex of B-vitamins	Aids in cell growth & development, metabolism, & use of other B-vitamins; helps relieve muscle pain, prevent hair loss (Under good conditions, our body manufactures some biotin.)	Dose: 100-300 mcg / day (No RDA)	None known
Choline (water soluble) Part of the complex of B-vitamins.	Maintains proper nerve transmissions, brain function & memory, liver function, gall bladder, and hormone production (Under good conditions, our body manufactures some choline.)	Dose: 400-900 mg / day (No RDA)	"Fishy" odor to body, diarrhea, depression
Folic Acid (water soluble) Part of the complex of B-vitamins	Maintains healthy blood; prevents birth defects; protects DNA/RNA; strengthens immunity; feeds the brain; eases breathing and memory problems Oral contraceptives increase need for folic acid. Our body manufactures some folic acid.	Dose: 400 mcg / day Toxic: 3000-15,000 mcg /day (No RDA)	Nausea, sleep disturbances, irritability, conflicts with epilepsy and schizophrenia drugs, inhibits zinc uptake

Inositol (water soluble) Part of the complex of B-vitamins	Reduces cholesterol; prevents hardening of arteries; needed for hair growth; metabolizes fats and cholesterol; has calming effects; prevents irritability and mood swings. (Under good conditions our body manufactures some inositol.)	Dose: Unknown Toxic: Unknown	
Vitamin C Ascorbic Acid (water soluble)	Fights infection; necessary for metabolism and collagen formation; speeds healing, helps absorb iron, lower cholesterol and blood pressure, lessens bruising	RDA Dose: 60-80 mg / day Toxic: 30,000 mg / day by mouth	Diarrhea; increases pain perception; masks copper deficiency; kidney stones
Vitamin D Ergocalciferol and Cholecalciferol (oil soluble)	Regulates calcium and phosphorus use; needed for bones and teeth; promotes regular heartbeat; enhances immunity; necessary for thyroid function, good eyes, weight loss & healthy appetite	RDA Dose: 200-400 iu / day Toxic: can be as low as 1000 iu/day in some, and 1,000,000 iu / day in others.	Nausea, thirst, vomiting, headache, confusion, delirium, coma, shock & death, kidney failure, osteoporosis, calcification of organs & blood vessels
Vitamin E Tocopherol (oil soluble)	An antioxidant that improves circulation, tissue repair; needed for fat metabolism; lowers cholesterol & blood pressure; works as skin/hair conditioner; keeps nerves healthy; helps prevent cancer and heart disease	RDA Dose: 30 iu / day Toxic: 600iu/day in a few, and 2000 iu/day in most others.	Severe weakness and fatigue; gas, diarrhea, hives, chapped lips
Vitamin K (oil soluble)	Needed for bone repair and formation; production of prothrombin, healthy liver, resistance to infection, and longevity; protects against cancers that form inside organs	RDA Dose: unknown Toxic: unknown	Flushing; toxic to fetus in utero
	Glandulars		
Raw Adrenal	Supports adrenals, helps the body manage stress, is useful in diabetes		
Raw Brain	Supports brain function, memory		
Raw Heart	Supports the heart and the heart-lung relationship		
Raw Kidney	Supports the kidney		

Raw Liver	Supports the liver, helps make liver enzymes		
Raw Lung	Supports the lungs and lung function in asthma, allergies, cancers, etc.		
Raw Mammary Gland	Supports the breast in cases of breast cancer		
Raw Ovary	Supports the ovaries in cases of PMS, hysterectomy, cysts, etc.		
Raw Pancreas	Supports the pancreas, helps the body produce digestive and other enzymes		
Raw Parathyroid	Supports the parathyroid glands, manages calcium metabolism, helps prevent loss of hair, gruff voice, etc.		
Raw Pituitary	Supports the pituitary function, keeps the body fluidified		
Raw Spleen	Supports the spleen and making of new red blood cells		
Raw Thymus	Supports the thymus and the entire immune system		
Raw Thyroid	Supports the thyroid and the dozens of functions it has, inc. diet, weight, osteoporosis, etc.		
Raw Orchic	Supports the testicles and helps maintain normal function in males		

Enzymes	*Function*	*Source*	
Amylase	Works with other enzymes to digest sugars and starches, improves the absorption of nutrients from food.	Aspergillus	
Bromelain	Helps reduce swelling and inflammation of joints, injuries; aids in amelioration of burns, thrombosis, cellulitis, and skin infections; accelerates the healing of bruises, abrasions, and contusions	Pineapple stem	
Chymotrypsin	Helps the immune system identify tumors and can dissolve the fibrin covering of cancers; reduces the blood stickiness that helps tumors/growths spread	Animal organs	

Lipase	Works with pancreatin to digest fats, improve the function of the pancreas and improve digestion overall	Aspergillus	
Pancreatin	An important family of enzymes in the digestion process. Improves digestion in older people	Animal organs	
Papain	Reduces inflammation and stimulates Tumor Necrosis Factor (TNF) which destroys growths. Destroys bacteria associated with stomach disorders like gastritis and ulcers.	Papaya	
Protease	Works with other enzymes to digest proteins and improve digestion overall.	Several sources	
Rutin	A free-radical scavenger that also destroys viruses and numerous bacteria. Rutin is a repairman of varicose veins and capillaries.	Several plants	
Trypsin	Accelerates healing of injuries, assists your immune system, reduces blood stickiness from phlebitis, emboli, and thromboses. Also dissolves the fibrin covering on cancer cells.	Ox pancreas	
	Exercise		
The Five Rites of the Fountain of Youth by Peter Kelder	Ancient yoga-like exercises out of Tibet that stimulate the endocrine system, reverse aging, and create an amazing amount of physical, mental, and emotional energy that lasts for approximately 2 ½ days	Do the entire set at least 3-4 times a week. Do up to 21 of each rite.	
Yoga	Any good yoga tape or instructor can provide you with guidance in performing the stretches this system offers.	20-30 minutes each day is ideal	
Walking	Go outside and walk – not fast – but at a good pace, with arms swinging naturally.	Walk at least twice a week for 30 min.	
Free weights	Use to maintain upper body strength	15-20 min. 3 times/wk	

Affirmations, Imagery, and Dreams

It is very important to maintain a positive attitude and engage in practical thinking. Don't panic!! If you take a turn for the worse, stop and assess what is happening. Think back over the past four to seven days and ask yourself what you might have done to trigger the situation as it is, or what the body is trying to accomplish. It could be a useful healing crisis manufactured by the body to accomplish its own goals. Trust your body. It knows what it is doing. Listen to the signals and pay attention to the messages it sends you.

Affirmations are also important. Come up with at least one statement or thought that affirms your self, your healing, your body, your courage, or some other aspect of the healing journey you are on. Write it down and post it where you can see it every day. When a specific fear comes up, face the fear until you get to the bottom of it to unearth its core belief about yourself or life. Usually the belief is simply not true. Then create an affirmation that specifically counters the belief and soothes the fear.

Examples of this might be your abject fear of dying...or of worsening pain...of serious scars...of being disabled...of your resistance to what you are experiencing...of embarrassment over your situation... or the belief that an infection (or perhaps a cancer) cannot be healed. Affirmations that counter these might be something like "I am alive, living in the light, and loving it" or "I am able to put my attention anywhere I want it to be" or "My body knows how to heal itself perfectly and I am listening to it and doing what it needs me to do" or "I am excited about the healing journey I'm on and ready to do whatever is needed for good health" or "My body and I can figure out how to heal anything, and we have the patience and persistence to do so."

If you are seriously ill, spend time at least once a day doing some healing imagery. This can be anything from seeing yourself going into the problem area, cleaning it out, and removing the difficulty to imagining you are constructing an entirely new body, to visualizing yourself doing something you have always wanted to do in a setting in which you're perfectly healthy.

In your mind, pick out several symbols of your own healing. For instance, give yourself the instruction that every time you notice a particular item, hear a certain song, or notice a ceetain color, it will be a reminder of your whole, healed Self. Then ask your body/mind system to bring the symbols to your attention as often as possible so that you are constantly reminded and reassured of the healing processes taking place inside you. When one of your healing symbols comes to your attention, be sure to thank yourself for noticing it, then spend a moment or two picturing yourself as completely healed and functioning normally.

Pay attention to your dreams, especially healing dreams or dreams that bring deeply buried issues or a reassuring awareness into consciousness. Write them down and study them until you have grasped the subtleties of their message to you. If they point to an action or a direction, take that action or go in that direction. Use the awareness to deepen your healing abilities.

Affirmations spontaneously created right now:

Recent Dreams that had an impact on you:

Daydreams that recur and seem to have significance:

Intuition

Pay attention to the miscellaneous thoughts and intuitions that cross your mind. When a thought comes to you more than once or twice, there is often some valuable reason for it. Pay special attention to those thoughts that take the form, "Maybe I should..." or "This doesn't feel right... I should stop doing (or eating) this..."

Above all, live as if you are going to live. Each day is a decision point in life!

Support

In your efforts to change your life and embark on a healing journey, who will nurture and support you? It's really important to have at least one person who will encourage and push you to keep going with your healing program. Ideally, that would be a spouse or family member. A true friend is also a good choice. Name at least two people who might be willing to support your healing program.

Support Person #1:

Support Person #2:

Obstacles

Are you willing to take the time needed for healing? If not – Why? What is in the way? Nothing is more important than your health. Note here your biggest obstacles, whether physical, mental, emotional, or spiritual, and evaluate your willingness to take the time you need for healing.

Physical: (e.g. money, relationships)

Mental: (e.g. uncertainty, not enough information)

Emotional: (e.g. self-worth, fear of what you might have to do)

Spiritual: (e.g. what will this mean about you or your life?)

Other obstacles I would have to deal with:

Your Space

Is your physical space set up to promote a healing lifestyle? Take a look around your kitchen. You may need new, updated, or additional small appliances in your kitchen. Jot down the most obvious things you would have to move, install, change, rearrange, or purchase and set up to make your kitchen work as one of the major support centers of a healing home.

Then take a look around your entire house, especially the bathroom, bedroom, even the yard. You might need space for exercise, a healing bathroom, a meditation space, an herb garden or small vegetable garden for fresh organic foods at least several months out of the year, different colors in your bedroom or living room, or some other arrangement. What would you do first? Second? Third? Jot down the changes needed in your space arrangements.

Kitchen:

Bathroom:

Bedroom:

Living Room:

Yard:

Other rooms:

Sleep and Rest

I need _____ hours of sleep each day/night in order to get the rest needed for healing.

Normal sleep habits can suffer when you are ill, but it is very important to get extra sleep *and* rest. Sleep is sleep. Rest is rest. Sleep can be rest, but rest is not necessarily sleep. Therefore, if you aren't sleeping well, it becomes all the more important to rest.

During a recent period of extreme stress and overwork, I found myself waking up in the night. At first, I was waking at 4:30 am, soon it was 3:30 am. Before long I was going to bed at midnight and waking at 1:30 am after only an hour or so of sleep. I'm not a napper and couldn't sleep during the day, so it was clear to me I was running on adrenaline. Since I couldn't see any way out of the situation, I ignored the sleeplessness until I crashed and burned. Of course, then I needed almost a year to repair and rebuild.

If you aren't getting enough sleep, it becomes doubly important to just rest. To rest is to relax, and while it can mean lying down for a while, it can also mean doing something that brings you great pleasure and doesn't require interaction with others. This can be going to the beach to watch a sunrise or a sunset, perhaps a walk in the woods, time to daydream, read, paint, fish, cross-stitch, putter in your shop, listen to music, or enjoy any light activity that brings a sense of renewal, peace, and satisfaction.

If you aren't sleeping, try a cup of melatonin tea about an hour before bedtime. If you're already in bed tossing and turning, do some very deep breathing as follows.

1. Using your diaphragm to pull upwards on the bottom of your lungs, exhaust as much air from your lungs as you can, then count to 4 slowly before breathing in.

2. Breathe in (through your nose, if you can) as deeply as possible, expanding your belly, your back, your sides, and your entire body as you completely fill your lungs. See the breath entering you as golden-pink light that goes directly to the place in you that needs healing. Count to 8 slowly, then release the air slowly, envisioning that you are exhaling the illness and all of its symptoms.

3. When all the air is exhausted, pull up on your diaphragm at the very end of the exhale to exhaust the last drop of air and empty yourself completely. Count to 4 slowly.

4. Breathe in again, relaxing the diaphragm, and filling your lungs and your entire body as in Step 2. When filled with golden-pink light, count to 8 slowly, and then release the air through pursed lips.

5. Exhaust all of the air, pulling up on your diaphragm at the end of the exhale to get all the air out of the lower lobes of the lungs. When empty, count to 4 slowly.

6. Repeat until you have done somewhere between 10 and 20 deep breaths. Then go to sleep. You will probably sleep deeply and well. Oxygen is a great relaxer!

Intuitive Checklist

At this point, after reading through the entire book, you should have at least some idea of the foods, detox procedures, minerals, vitamins, glandulars, enzymes, and exercises that make up a healing program. If you've also read the first part of this appendix, you have considered affirmations, support issues, personal obstacles, and the physical changes that might be needed in your living space.

Now, without reviewing the book, and working solely on the basis of intuition, check off those procedures, supplements, foods, exercises, and changes that the all-knowing part of you feels would be important for you to include in your personal healing program.

Fasting:

      Water Fast   _____

      Juice Fast   _____

      Herbal Tea Fast   _____

Exercise:

      Fountain of Youth   _____

      Yoga   _____

      Walking   _____

      Physical labor   _____

Daily Detox:

      Coffee enema   _____

      Mustard Foot Soak   _____

      Castor Oil Pack   _____

      Clay for Parasites   _____

      Salt and Soda Bath   _____

Water:

      64 oz/day   _____

      128 oz/day   _____

Weekly Detox:
    Chelation – EDTA   _____
    1-day Juice Fast   _____
    3-day Juice Fast   _____
    5-day Juice Fast   _____
    3-day Water Fast   _____
    5-day Water Fast   _____
    8-day Water Fast   _____
    Castor/Olive Oil Sweat   _____
Monthly or Annual Detox:
    Liver Flush   _____
    Colon Sweep   _____
    The Purge   _____
    Chelation – DMPS   _____
    Full Parasite Program   _____
Supplements:
    Amino Acids   _____
    The Basic 6 Minerals   _____
    Vitamin A   _____
    Vitamin B-Complex   _____
    Vitamin C   _____
    Vitamin D   _____
    Vitamin E   _____
    Specific, extra
      vitamins/supplements   _____
      that you know about   _____
      or have used with   _____
      success & which   _____
      might be useful   _____

    _____
    Digestive Enzymes   _____
    Pancreas Enzymes   _____
Additional Useful Supplements:
    Liquid Trace Minerals   _____
    Sulfur/MSM   _____
    Copper   _____
    Boron   _____
    Silica   _____
    Silver   _____
    Gold   _____
    Selenium   _____

Germanium   _____
Manganese   _____
Iodine   _____
Glucosamine   _____
Gingko Biloba   _____
Saw Palmetto   _____
Hawthorne Berry   _____
DHEA   _____
Bilberry   _____
Milk Thistle   _____
Nettle   _____
RNA/DNA   _____
Bentonite clay   _____
Primrose Oil   _____
Borage Oil   _____
Black Currant Seed Oil   _____
Glandulars:
Raw Adrenal   _____
Raw Brain   _____
Raw Heart   _____
Raw Kidney   _____
Raw Liver   _____
Raw Lung   _____
Raw Mammary   _____
Raw Ovary   _____
Raw Parathryoid   _____
Raw Pancreas   _____
Raw Pituitary   _____
Raw Spleen   _____
Raw Thymus   _____
Raw Thyroid   _____
Glandular Complex   _____
Organic Foods:
Beef   _____
Chicken   _____
Lamb   _____
Pork   _____
Fish   _____
Milk   _____
Buttermilk   _____
Butter   _____

Yogurt   _____

Cheese   _____

Eggs   _____

Flaxseed Oil   _____

Hempseed Oil   _____

Raw Vegetables   _____

Raw carrot juice   _____

Raw fruits   _____

Raw fruit juice   _____

Raw almonds   _____

Freshly ground whole
  wheat breads   _____

14-Grain Cereal   _____

Breads made from spelt,
  oats, rye, etc.   _____

Organic wine (red)   _____

Green tea   _____

Black tea   _____

Herb teas   _____

Foods to reduce, temporarily avoid, or compensate for:

  Coffee (more than 2 c/day) _____

  Cigarettes (consider growing
    your own tobacco)   _____

  Alcohol   _____

Foods to avoid forever:

  White flour products   _____

  White sugar products   _____

  Soy   _____

  Margarine   _____

  Polyunsaturated fats   _____

  Foods in bottles, boxes,
    and cans   _____

Once you have used your intuition to check off the things you think would be helpful in your healing program, combine it with your common sense and logic to decide what you will actually do, where you will begin, etc. When your healing program is under way, refer back to the checklist from time to time, as there will be things you forgot to implement, as well as new intuitions to guide you.

In closing, it should be obvious that you will have to make some lifestyle changes during the time you are healing. A friend of mine with cancer did not want to bother with the detox routines that are so critical for liver and tissue support. He said he didn't have time for that sort of thing and turned his nose up at the coffee enemas. He only wanted to change what he ate. I argued to no avail. Now he not only doesn't have time, he isn't alive to worry about it.

Educate yourself to do the majority of your own healing. Take time to reconnect with Mother Nature and the soil. Take time to find good sources of high-nutrition food and do the detox routines. Develop the strength to change your life. As I have pointed out before, it is not your job to heal your body. Your body will heal itself. Your job is to figure out how to support and nurture the healing process going on within you.

Act! Even if you have some doubts. You will learn as you go along. I can't count the number of people who thought it was hopeless in the beginning when it wasn't. They waited until it was too late, then frantically tried to take action. Don't stand around waiting for a magic button or a magic pill.

On the other hand, I have seen miracles and sometimes think it is never too late. Just remember this...you are a body/mind system with individualized needs. Begin filling them wisely and well in accord with how Nature intended, and you will heal. Whether the miracle takes 20 minutes or 20 months is not important. What is important is that you take action at all levels – physically, mentally, emotionally, and spiritually.

May your efforts be blessed with success, everlasting good health, and wisdom. ❖

Appendix B
Suggested Reading and References

THE FOLLOWING is a very partial alphabetical listing of books that would be good to have in your library. Everyone who intends to heal either the self or anyone else in the family should maintain a small library of books that contains a combination of accurate knowledge, hands-on techniques, reference material, old and new wisdom. Hopefully these references will also impart a level of sensitivity and awareness to people, plants, animals, and the Earth. **I have put an asterisk next to those I consider to be basic, necessary references and that should be on every family bookshelf.** The rest are all important in one way or another and are critical to a full understanding of the issues currently facing us today if we want to live and be well.

A Promise Made, A Promise Kept: One Son's Quest for the Cause and Cure of Diabetes by Dr. James Chappell, DC, ND, PhD, MH; BL Publications, Detroit Lakes, MN, 2005. ISBN 1-890766-3152995.

Biomimicry by Janine M. Benyus; Wm. Morrow and Co. Inc., New York, 1997. ISBN 0-688-13691-5.

* *Dr. Wright's Guide to Healing With Nutrition* by Jonathan V. Wright, MD; Keats Publishing Inc., 1989. ISBN 0-87983-530-3.

Empty Harvest by Dr. Bernard Jensen and Mark Anderson; Avery Publishing Group, Inc., Garden City Park, NY, 1990. ISBN 0-89529-558-X.

* *Encyclopedia of Natural Medicine* by Michael Murray, ND and Joseph Pizzorno, ND; Prima Publishing, Rocklin, CA, 1998. ISBN 0-7615-1157-1.

* *Enzyme Nutrition: The Food Enzyme Concept* by Dr. Edward Howell; Avery Publishing Group, Inc. 1985. ISBN 0-89529-300-5.

* *Fasting Can Save Your Life* by Herbert M. Shelton; American Natural Hygiene Society, 1991. ISBN 0-914532-23-5.

Fats That Heal, Fats That Kill by Udo Erasmus; Alive Books, Burnaby, BC, Canada, 1997. ISBN 0-920470-38-6.

Fit For Life by Harvey & Marilyn Diamond; Warner Books Inc. 1985. ISBN 0-446-30015-2.

From Fatigued to Fantastic by Jacob Teitelbaum, MD; Avery Books, New York, NY, 2001. ISBN 1-58333-097-6.

How To Get Well by Paavo Airola, PhD; Health Plus Publishers, 1974. ISBN 0-932090-03-6.

In The Absence of The Sacred by Jerry Mander; Sierra Club Books, San Francisco, CA, 1992. ISBN 0-87156-509-9.

* *It's All In Your Head* by Hal S. Huggins, DDS; MS, Avery Publishing, NY, 1993. ISBN 0-89529-550-4.

Living Water by Olof Alexandersson; Gateway Books, Bath, United Kingdom, 1996. ISBN 0-946551-57-X.

Living Cuisine by Rene Loux Underkoffler; Avery Publishing, New York, NY, 2003. ISBN 1-58333-171-9.

* *Nourishing Traditions Cookbook* by Sally Fallon; ProMotion Publishing, San Diego, CA, 1995. ISBN 1-887314-15-6.

Nutrition and Mental Illness: An Orthomolecular Approach to Balancing Body Chemistry by Carl C. Pfeiffer, PhD, MD; Healing Arts Press, Rochester, VT, 1987. ISBN 0-89281-226-5.

* *Nutrition and Physical Degeneration* by Weston A. Price, DDS.; Keats Publishing, 1989. ISBN 0-87983-502-8.

Nutrition and The Mind by Gary Null, PhD; Four Walls Eight Windows Press, New York, NY, 1995. ISBN 1-56858-021-5.

* *Our Earth, Our Cure* by Raymond Dextreit, translated and edited by Michel Abehsera; Citadel Press Book, Carols Publishing Group Edition, New York, 1993. ISBN 0-8065-1013-7.

Permaculture by Bill Mollison; Tagari Press; Tyalgum, NSW, Australia, 1996. ISBN 0-908228-01-5.

* *Prescription for Nutritional Healing, 2nd Edition* by James F. Balch, MD & Phyllis A. Balch, CNC; Avery Publishing Group, 1997. ISBN 0-90529-727-2.

* *Prescription for Herbal Healing* by Phyllis A. Balch, CNC; Avery Publishing, a member of Penguin Putnam, Inc. New York, NY; 2002. ISBN 0-89529-869-4.

Robes – A Book of Coming Changes by Penny Kelly; Lily Hill Publishing, Lawton, MI. ISBN 0-9632934-2-7.

Solved: The Riddle of Illness by Stephen E. Langer, MD and James F. Scheer; Keats Publishing, CA. ISBN 0-658-00293-7.

* *Stolen Harvest* by Vandana Shiva; South End Press, Cambridge, MA, 1999. ISBN 0-89608-607-0.

* *Sugar Blues* by William Dufty; Warner Books Inc., NY, 1993. ISBN 0-556-34312-9.

* *The Ancient Secret of The Fountain of Youth* by Peter Kelder; Doubleday, NY, 1998. ISBN 0-385-49162-X.

The China Study by T. Colin Campbell, PhD and Thomas M. Campbell II; BenBella Books; Dallas, TX, 2006. ISBN 978-1932100-66-2.

* *The Healing Power of Herbs* by Michael T. Murray, ND; Prima Publishing, Rocklin, CA, 1995. ISBN 1-55958-700-8.

The Right Dose: How to Take Vitamins & Minerals Safely by Patricia Hausman, MS; Ballantine Book, NY, 1992. ISBN 0-345-335877-5.

The Rodale Book of Composting, ed. Deborah L. Martin & Grace Gershuny; Rodale Press, 1992. ISBN 0-87857-991-5.

The Secret Life of Plants by Christopher Bird and Peter Tompkins; Harper Collins Publishers, New York, NY, 2002. ISBN 0-60-091587-0

The Secrets of The Soil by Christopher Bird and Peter Tompkins; Harper & Row Publishers, New York, NY, 1989. ISBN 0-06-091968-X.

Tissue Cleansing Through Bowel Management by Bernard Jensen, DC; Bernard Jenzen Enterprises, Escondido, CA, 1981. No ISBN. www.bernardjensen.com.

Vitality Foods for Health & Fitness by Pierre Jean Cousin & Kirsten Hartvig, Duncan Baird Publishers, London, UK, 2002. ISBN 1-903296-88-9.

Water: For Health, for Healing, for Life by F. Batmanghelidg, MD; Warner Books, New York, NY, 2003. ISBN 0-446-69074-0.

What Your Doctor May Not Tell You About Menopause: The Breakthrough Book on Natural Progesterone by John R. Lee, MD; Warner Books, New York, NY, 1996; ISBN 0-446-67144-4.

* *Your Body's Many Cries for Water* by F. Batmanghelidj, MD; Global Health Solutions, Inc, Falls Church, VA, 1995; ISBN 0-9629942-3-5.

❖

Index

A

A. F. Tredgold, 26
Abehsera, Michel, 226
Aborigines, Australian, 22
abscessed jaws, 31
absorbtion of food, 52
acid environment, 174
actinomycetes, 42
ADHD, 34, 105, 199
adrenal glands, 34
adrenals, 177
adrenocorticotropic hormone, 194
Affirmations, 279
Africa, East and Central, 21
aggressive behavior, 199
agriculture, chemical, 73
agriculture, corporate-style, 74
AIDS, 219
Airola, PhD ND, Paavo, 134
Alanine, 184
alarm, 194
Albrecht, William, 73
alcoholism, 33, 199
 Stornoway Island, 20
Alcoholism, 200
alkaline environment, 174
allergies, 34
allergies and milk, 99
allergies, killer, 35
allergy bull's-eyes, 101
allopathic doctors
 and treatment, 207
allopathic medicine, 208
Allopathic medicine
 as rescue, 12
allopathy and responsibility for patient,
 11
aloe vera compress, 216
Alzheimer's, 199
American Medical Association, 10
Amino acids, 181, 182
amino acids in meat, 93
amino acids in plants, 44
amylase, 175

anorexia, 199
antennae, insect, 48
antibiotic-resistant drugs, 170
antibiotics, 89
antioxidants and polyunsaturated fats,
 112
appliances, small, 282
Arabic people, 118
Arachidonic Acid, 112
Arginine, 184
arsenic, 45
art as household items, 195
artesian springs, 60
arthritis, 2, 33, 179
 in 6-yr.-olds, 35
artificial insemination, 35
Asparagine, 184
aspartame, 168
Aspartic acid, 184
asthma and glandulars, 178
asthmatics, 34
asylums, 26
atherosclerosis, 110
atomic bomb project, 230
ATP, 250
autism, 199
autistic children, 201
auxones, 84

B

bacon fat, 113
bacteria and disease, 95
Balch C.N.C., Phyllis, 185
Bang's Disease, 99
Bardsey Island, 20
Barley, 116
beauty in America, 29
Bechamp, Pierre, 95
beef tallow, 113
beef that shrinks, 91
beef, tenderizing, 91
beet root, 175
believing in something, 206
Bentonite clay, 227

T

About The Author

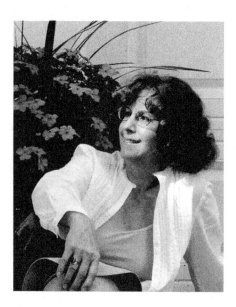

Penny Kelly is the owner of Lily Hill Farm & Learning Center in southwest Michigan where she writes and teaches classes in *Developing and Using Intuition, Organic Gardening,* and *Getting Well Again Naturally.* She does nutritional consultations, maintains a large spiritual counseling practice, and raises cows and chickens as well as organic vegetables and fruits.

She is deeply involved in helping to organize the Community Gardening movement in Kalamazoo and Battle Creek, MI, and is working to create a regional food system and food council in southwest Michigan.

Penny holds a degree in Humanistic Studies from Wayne State University, a degree in Naturopathic Medicine from Clayton College of Natural Health, and is currently working toward her Ph.D. in nutrition from the American Holistic College of Nutrition.

In addition to this book, Penny has written four other books: *The Evolving Human, The Elves of Lily Hill Farm, Robes: A Book of Coming Changes,* and *Consciousness and Energy, Vol. 1.* She has also co-authored 14 books for the Ultimate Destiny Success System and is currently at work on *Consciousness and Energy, Vol. 2,* due out in 2010.

Visit her website at www.pennykelly.com.

CPSIA information can be obtained at www.ICGtesting.com
Printed in the USA
BVOW08s2043290116

434468BV00002B/150/P